Critical Reflections on Stanley Hauerwas' Theology of Disability: Disabling Society, Enabling Theology

Critical Reflections on Stanley Hauerwas' Theology of Disability: Disabling Society, Enabling Theology has been co-published simultaneously as *Journal of Religion, Disability & Health*, Volume 8, Numbers 3/4 2004.

The *Journal of Religion, Disability & Health*™ Monographic "Separates"

(formerly the *Journal of Religion in Disability & Rehabilitation* series)*

Below is a list of "separates," which in serials librarianship means a special issue simultaneously published as a special journal issue or double-issue *and* as a "separate" hardbound monograph. (This is a format which we also call a "DocuSerial.")

"Separates" are published because specialized libraries or professionals may wish to purchase a specific thematic issue by itself in a format which can be separately cataloged and shelved, as opposed to purchas - ing the journal on an on-going basis. Faculty members may also more easily consider a "separate" for classroom adoption.

"Separates" are carefully classified separately with the major book jobbers so that the journal tie-in can be noted on new book order slips to avoid duplicate purchasing.

You may wish to visit Haworth's website at . . .

http://www.HaworthPress.com

. . . to search our online catalog for complete tables of contents of these separates and related publications.

You may also call 1-800-HAWORTH (outside US/Canada: 607-722-5857), or Fax 1-800-895-0582 (outside US/Canada: 607-771-0012), or e-mail at:

docdelivery@haworthpress.com

Critical Reflections on Stanley Hauerwas' Theology of Disability: Disabling Society, Enabling Theology, edited by John Swinton, PhD (Vol. 8, No. 3/4, 2004). *"AN EXCELLENT AND LONG-NEEDED RESOURCE . . . This work will not only continue the ongoing discussion among those specializing in the theology of disability in general and disability related to intellectual development in particular, but will also serve to bring disability into the mainline of contemporary theological discussion." (Kerry H. Wynn, PhD, Director, Learning Enrichment Center Southeast Missouri State University)*

Voices in Disability and Spirituality from the Land Down Under: From Outback to Outfront, edited by Rev. Dr. Christopher Newell, PhD, and Rev. Andy Calder (Vol. 8, No. 1/2, 2004). *"In recent years disability theology has emerged alongside Black theology and womens' theology as a new genre seeking to express the concerns of people whose experience has often been marginalized. This collection is A SIGNIFICANT AUSTRALIAN CONTRIBUTION TO THIS GROWING LITERATURE. The early explorers named Australia 'the south land of the Holy Spirit.' (John M. Hull, PhD, Hon DTheol, Professor Emeritus of Religious Education, University of Birmingham, England; Author of* On Sight and Insight *and* In the Beginning There was Darkness)

Graduate Theological Education and the Human Experience of Disability, edited by Robert C. Anderson (Vol. 7, No. 3, 2003). *"A comprehensive overview of theological education and disability. . . . Concise and well written. . . . Offers rich theological insights and abundant practical advice. I strongly recommend this volume as a key introduction to this important emerging topic in theological education." (Rev. John W. Crossin, PhD, OSFS, Executive Director, Washington Theological Consortium)*

The Pastoral Voice of Robert Perske, edited by William C. Gaventa, Jr., MDiv, and David L. Coulter, MD (Vol. 7, No. 1/2, 2003). *"Must reading for seminary students and clinincal program directors. Pastors, providers, and parents concerned with persons suffering from cognitive, intellectual, and developmental disabilities will find these vigorous testimonies readable, timely, fresh, and inspiring despite having been written more than 30 years ago." (Barbara J. Lampe, JD, Executive Director, National Apostolate for Inclusion Ministry)*

Spirituality and Intellectual Disability: International Perspectives on the Effect of Culture and Religion on Healing Body, Mind, and Soul, edited by William C. Gaventa, Jr., MDiv, and David L. Coulter, MD (Vol. 5, No. 2/3, 2001). *"Must reading . . . perspectives from many faiths and cultures on the spiritual needs and gifts of people with mental retardation." (Ginny Thornburgh, EdM, Religion and Disability Program, National Organization on Disability, Washington, DC)*

The Theological Voice of Wolf Wolfensberger, edited by William C. Gaventa, MDiv, and David L. Coulter, MD (Vol. 4, No. 2/3, 2001). *This thought-provoking volume presents Wolfensberger's challenging, outrageous, and inspiring ideas on the theological significance of disabilities, including the problem with wheelchair access ramps in churches, the meaning of suffering, and the spiritual gifts of the mentally retarded.*

A Look Back: The Birth of the Americans With Disabilities Act, edited by Robert C. Anderson, MDiv (Vol. 2, No. 4, 1996).* *Takes you to the unique moment in American history when persons of many different backgrounds and with different disabilities united to press Congress for full recognition and protection of their rights as American citizens.*

Pastoral Care of the Mentally Disabled: Advancing Care of the Whole Person, edited by Sally K. Severino, MD, and Reverend Richard Liew, PhD (Vol. 1, No. 2, 1994).* *"A great book for theologians with a refreshing dogma-free approach; thought provoking for physiotherapists and all other human beings!" (The Chartered Society of Physiotherapy)*

Critical Reflections on Stanley Hauerwas' Theology of Disability: Disabling Society, Enabling Theology

John Swinton, PhD
Editor

Critical Reflections on Stanley Hauerwas' Theology of Disability: Disabling Society, Enabling Theology has been co-published simultaneously as *Journal of Religion, Disability & Health*, Volume 8, Numbers 3/4 2004.

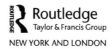

Routledge
Taylor & Francis Group

NEW YORK AND LONDON

First Published by

The Haworth Pastoral Press, 10 Alice Street, Binghamton, NY 13904-1580 USA

The Haworth Pastoral Press is an imprint of The Haworth Press, Inc., 10 Alice Street, Binghamton, NY 13904-1580 USA.

Transferred to Digital Printing 2008 by Routledge
270 Madison Ave, New York NY 10016
2 Park Square, Milton Park, Abingdon, Oxon, OX14 4RN

Critical Reflections on Stanley Hauerwas' Theology of Disability: Disabling Society, Enabling Theology has been co-published simultaneously as *Journal of Religion, Disability & Health*, Volume 8, Numbers 3/4 2004.

The development, preparation, and publication of this work has been undertaken with great care. However, the publisher, employees, editors, and agents of The Haworth Press and all imprints of The Haworth Press, Inc., including The Haworth Medical Press® and The Pharmaceutical Products Press®, are not responsible for any errors contained herein or for consequences that may ensue from use of materials or information contained in this work. Opinions expressed by the author(s) are not necessarily those of The Haworth Press, Inc.

Cover design by Jennifer Gaska

Library of Congress Cataloging-in-Publication Data

Critical Reflections on Stanley Hauerwas' Theology of Disability: Disabling Society, Enabling Theology / John Swinton, editor.
     p. cm.
"Co-published simultaneously as Journal of religion, disability & health, volume 8, numbers 3/4 2004"–T.p. verso.
    Includes bibliographical references and index.
    ISBN 0-7890-2721-6 (hard cover : alk. paper)–ISBN 0-7890-2722-4 (pbk. : alk. paper)
    1. Developmental disabilities–Religious aspects–Christianity. 2. Hauerwas, Stanley, 1940–Contributions in theology of developmental disabilities. I. Hauerwas, Stanley, 1940– II. Swinton, John, 1957– III. Journal of religion, disability & health.
BT732.4.C66 2005
261.8'324–dc22
                                                           2004017528

Publisher's Note
The publisher has gone to great lengths to ensure the quality of this reprint but points out that some imperfections in the original may be apparent.

Indexing, Abstracting & Website/Internet Coverage

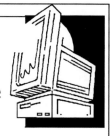

This section provides you with a list of major indexing & abstracting services and other tools for bibliographic access. That is to say, each service began covering this periodical during the year noted in the right column. Most Websites which are listed below have indicated that they will either post, disseminate, compile, archive, cite or alert their own Website users with research-based content from this work. (This list is as current as the copyright date of this publication.)

Abstracting, Website/Indexing Coverage . . . . Year When Coverage Began

- *Applied Social Sciences Index & Abstracts (ASSIA)*
  (Online: ASSI via Data-Star) (CDRom: ASSIA Plus)
  <http://www.csa.com> 1994

- *AURSI African Urban & Regional Science Index. A scholarly &*
  research index which synthesises & compiles all publications
  on urbanization & regional science in Africa within the world.
  Published annually 2004

- *CINAHL (Cumulative Index to Nursing & Allied Health*
  Literature), in print, EBSCO, and SilverPlatter, DataStar,
  and PaperChase (Support materials include Subject Heading List,
  Database Search Guide, and instructional video)
  <http://www.cinahl.com> 1999

- *e-psyche, LLC <http://www.e-psyche.net>* 2002

- *Educational Research Abstracts (ERA) (online database)*
  <http://www.tandf.co.uk/era>. 2003

- *Family & Society Studies Worldwide*
  <http://www.nisc.com>. 1996

- *Family Index Database*
  <http://www.familyscholar.com>. 2003

- *Human Resources Abstracts (HRA)* 1994

- *IBZ International Bibliography of Periodical Literature*
  <http://www.saur.de> 2001

(continued)

Special Bibliographic Notes related to special journal issues (separates) and indexing/abstracting:

- indexing/abstracting services in this list will also cover material in any "separate" that is co-published simultaneously with Haworth's special thematic journal issue or DocuSerial. Indexing/abstracting usually covers material at the article/chapter level.
- monographic co-editions are intended for either non-subscribers or libraries which intend to purchase a second copy for their circulating collections.
- monographic co-editions are reported to all jobbers/wholesalers/approval plans. The source journal is listed as the "series" to assist the prevention of duplicate purchasing in the same manner utilized for books-in-series.
- to facilitate user/access services all indexing/abstracting services are encouraged to utilize the co-indexing entry note indicated at the bottom of the first page of each article/chapter/contribution.
- this is intended to assist a library user of any reference tool (whether print, electronic, online, or CD-ROM) to locate the monographic version if the library has purchased this version but not a subscription to the source journal.
- individual articles/chapters in any Haworth publication are also available through the Haworth Document Delivery Service (HDDS).

Critical Reflections on Stanley Hauerwas' Theology of Disability: Disabling Society, Enabling Theology

CONTENTS

ABOUT THE EDITOR

John Swinton, PhD, BD, RNM, RNMH, is Professor in Practical Theology and Pastoral Care in the School of Divinity, History, and Philosophy at the University of Aberdeen, Scotland. He has researched and published extensively on practical theology, mental health, spirituality and human well-being, and the theology of disability. His books include *Spirituality in Mental Health Care: Rediscovering a Forgotten Dimension*; *The Spiritual Dimension of Pastoral Care: Practical Theology in a Multidisciplinary Context* (edited with David Willows); and *From Bedlam to Shalom: Towards a Practical Theology of Human Nature, Interpersonal Relationships, and Mental Health Care*. Dr. Swinton is an ordained minister in the Church of Scotland.

Foreword:
A Doctor's Debt to Stanley Hauerwas

SUMMARY. The author acknowledges his debt to Stanley Hauerwas by describing how Hauerwas' writing has influenced his work as a pediatric neurologist. Hauerwas helped him to recognize that persons with intellectual disabilities have intrinsic value and that this value is based upon a spirituality shared with all of us. This recognition led the author to develop a clinical practice that is based on trying to see the world through the eyes of the person with a disability and to celebrate the wonder and value of the person's life. Hauerwas rightly emphasizes that the so-called question of personhood is fundamentally wrongheaded because no one's existence needs to be justified. This insight has helped the author confront the continuing problem of euthanasia for persons with disabilities and is reflected in the author's belief that peace-making (based on the recognition of the value of all persons regardless of disability) is the true answer to the problem of death-making (which is based on the devaluation of the lives of persons with disability). The author concludes by hoping that readers of this book will also find applications for Hauerwas' thinking in their own life and work. *[Article copies available for a fee from The Haworth Document Delivery Service: 1-800-HAWORTH. E-mail address: <docdelivery@haworthpress.com> Website: <http://www.HaworthPress.com> © 2004 by The Haworth Press, Inc. All rights reserved.]*

[Haworth co-indexing entry note]: "Foreword: A Doctor's Debt to Stanley Hauerwas." Coulter, David L. Co-published simultaneously in *Journal of Religion, Disability & Health* (The Haworth Pastoral Press, an imprint of The Haworth Press, Inc.) Vol. 8, No. 3/4, 2004, pp. xxi-xxvi; and: *Critical Reflections on Stanley Hauerwas' Theology of Disability: Disabling Society, Enabling Theology* (ed: John Swinton) The Haworth Pastoral Press, an imprint of The Haworth Press, Inc., 2004, pp. xiii-xviii. Single or multiple copies of this article are available for a fee from The Haworth Document Delivery Service [1-800-HAWORTH, 9:00 a.m. - 5:00 p.m. (EST). E-mail address: docdelivery@haworthpress.com].

xiii

KEYWORDS. Hauerwas, disability, personhood, medicine

I did not know Stanley Hauerwas when he was teaching at the University of Notre Dame in the 1960s. At the time I was an undergraduate at Notre Dame majoring in biology, thinking more about anatomy and physiology than about theology or the education of children with intellectual disabilities (what Hauerwas calls mental retardation). When my fellow students and I went off campus to visit the bars and pizza places that catered to Notre Dame students, we would pass the Saint Joseph Center for the Retarded where Professor Hauerwas was spending so much time. I often wondered what was going on in there. I knew that some students volunteered their time to work at the Center, but none of my friends did and I never found the time or inclination to volunteer myself. Little did I know at the time that 33 years later I would be writing this preface and explaining how much Professor Hauerwas' writings have influenced my work as a physician ever since.

I began to read Hauerwas in the 1980s when I was beginning my career as a pediatric neurologist, working with children with disabilities and their families on a daily basis and trying to figure out what was the right thing to do. I was the one who was called to the Neonatal Intensive Care Unit when a child was born with significant neurological disabilities and I was the one who had to explain the diagnosis and prognosis to the family. I realized that I needed to know a lot more about ethics than I had been taught in my medical training, which was not much. Secular philosophy and bioethics provided unsatisfying answers to the questions I was confronting. Perhaps because of my Catholic education at Notre Dame, I felt that there must be something more to the debate than this, something that would address the spiritual lives of persons with disabilities and the responsibilities we all have to live with them. So it was incredibly refreshing to discover that Hauerwas was thinking about the same issues and had a wealth of insight, experience and knowledge that could help me make sense of what I was doing every day.

Reading this collection of his papers now is like visiting an old friend who had been a cherished teacher and mentor in the past. Some of the papers in this collection are familiar to me from those days, but some I never saw because they were published in places I never read. And it is particularly refreshing to read his more recent papers which bring me up to date on what he is thinking about now. Perhaps one way I can pay tribute to Professor Hauerwas, the mentor I cherished but never met or knew personally, is to draw upon my own writing and experience to comment on his work and to show how much he has influenced my work as a doctor.

Hauerwas spends a lot of time trying to show that persons with intellectual disabilities are individuals with intrinsic value equal to those without disabilities. It is as if he starts by thinking that many people perceive an inequality, so he must show that this inequality is false. But what if we could start by thinking that there is a fundamental equality among all persons regardless of disability? In my clinical work, I developed a method for doing this that I called "the three ways of looking" (Coulter, 2001). I would sit down with a patient or family and try to get some idea of who they were as human beings and to try to see things through their eyes. I soon realized that I needed to share myself with them too and give them some idea of who I was. Thus the "first look" is to see the other person as an individual human being, and the "second look" is to see the other person as an individual like myself. If I know what it means for me to be alive and what I value in my own life, I can then try to understand what it means for the other person to be alive and what he or she values in his or her own life. And if I can do this, then I can value in the other person what I value most in my own life.

I came to realize that what we were sharing was our spirituality and that this did not depend on age, race, sex, wealth, or ability. Indeed, the "third look" is to see in each other the ground of all being and existence, the transcendence or divinity that informs our spirituality. This simple method was showing me that all persons are equal in value and human dignity, regardless of these various other characteristics, because they all possess intrinsic and universal spiritual worth. When this fundamental acceptance of the equality of all persons is our starting point, we do not need to justify the value or worth of persons with intellectual disabilities. We only need to see them as spiritual beings like us, which brings us to the same point Hauerwas emphasizes in his writing.

Thus my task as a physician and neurologist is to try to see the world through the eyes of persons with disabilities and to explain what I see to others, including families, friends, teachers, and therapists. My job is to try to understand what they are thinking and why they do what they do from a human perspective. If I can explain their behavior to others, then others will be better able to accept them as fully human persons too.

I have no doubt that reading Hauerwas during my formative years helped me to develop this clinical method and I readily acknowledge my debt to him. But Hauerwas goes further to emphasize the role each of us plays in the human community and our inextricable interdependence on each other, regardless of disability. He emphasizes that our role in the community is to live our own stories and through doing so, to live out the story of the Gospel. Our "value" to the community rests in these life stories, not in any "liberal" interpretation of autonomy or self-control. But what binds each of our life stories to each other?

Hauerwas may have the answer to this question. His concern about terminology and about "speaking for" persons with intellectual disabilities leads him to reflect on the nature of relationships within such a Christian community. In Chapter 1 he reflects on the wisdom of Jean Vanier and points out that there is no need to justify living in community with persons with intellectual disabilities because "you do not need to ask such questions about your friends." Some years ago I was listening to a professional debate about whether we should call persons with intellectual disabilities "patients" or "clients" or "consumers" or some such thing. I rose to suggest that perhaps the best term to use would be "friends." My professional colleagues did not like this idea, but I think Vanier and Hauerwas would have approved. Perhaps I got the idea from them.

The practical application of Hauerwas' thinking in my professional work shows up in other ways that are illustrated by the papers in this collection. In Chapter 2 he rightly emphasizes the respect parents deserve for loving and raising their children with disabilities. Twenty-five years of practice as a pediatric neurologist have taught me much the same thing. I am continually amazed by the strengths of families whose unceasing efforts are driven by their love for the child with a disability (Coulter, 2002). I tend to agree more with John O'Brien's response to this paper, but O'Brien is writing 25 years after Hauerwas gave the talk upon which Chapter 2 is based. This discussion illustrates another practical application of Hauerwas' thinking for us today. Normalization means many things, but today it means the right of persons with disabilities to live in the community of their choice and to experience the joys and friendships we all take for granted. Hauerwas rightly (if indirectly) emphasizes the need we all have for living together in community, which also means there can no longer be any justification for "putting someone away" in an institution.

I have spent a lot of time thinking about prevention of intellectual disability, mostly from a professional perspective (see Chapter 8 in American Association on Mental Retardation, 2002). Hauerwas addresses this topic in Chapter 5, which is reprinted from a book that I studied carefully when it was published. What he writes in the conclusion to this paper is the basis for the "third look" I described above. In the end, I have concluded that prevention should not be about reproductive choice, as Hauerwas implies. Rather, prevention should be about identifying ways that we can support individuals with disabilities and their families so that they can overcome limitations and enhance functioning to live more personally satisfying lives.

Hauerwas is vitally concerned about what it means to be a person, especially a person with an intellectual disability. To some extent this reflects the historical debate that was prominent at the time he was writing these papers, especially those in Chapters 6 and 7. I have struggled with this concept too, particularly in trying to figure out how to respond as a neurologist to patients with severe disabilities. Hauerwas is uncomfortable with the very question of personhood, and in these chapters he provides a way out of the dilemma. He suggests that the question itself is fundamentally wrong-headed because it implies that some human beings are persons and some are not, and all we need to do is figure a way to tell them apart. He suggests a different way of phrasing the question so that we focus on the disability of presence instead of the presence of disability. He uses Michael Bérubé's comment about accepting his disabled son, Jamie, "now that he is here" to show that we are all human creatures, created by God to "be here" and to be dependent on one another, just as Jamie is dependent on those around him. The presence that we all have "now that we are here" allows us to recognize the presents we all give to each other through our dependency on each other, including our ability and disability. Hauerwas returns to this point in his concluding response to the responses. He writes that the existence of persons with disabilities does not need to be justified (as, for example, by arguments about personhood) because no one's existence needs to be justified. "I exist, you exist, Jamie exists, turtles exist, the earth exists by the grace of God. The task is to learn to rejoice in our existence without resentment."

This is an important conclusion for those of us involved in bioethics because of the very real threats of euthanasia and devaluation of the lives of persons with disabilities. Hauerwas does not address this threat directly but he provides a way for us to respond by emphasizing the intrinsic dignity and worth of all persons who are created by God and now "are here" as valued members of a Christian community that depends on and cares for each other. As a physician and neurologist, I welcome this perspective and am able to apply it in my medical practice. Thank you, Professor Hauerwas, for helping me respond to these issues and showing me how to teach others to share this perspective.

I suspect I have not done justice to the wealth and depth of Hauerwas' theological arguments. I am, after all, a physician and not a theologian. I was given the opportunity to write this preface because I am the co-editor of *Journal of Religion, Disability & Health,* in which this collection appears. The mission of our *Journal* is to bridge clinical practice and spiritual supports for persons with disabilities. I hope that these remarks demonstrate one way to do this through the application of the theology of Stanley Hauerwas in my own clinical practice. Hauerwas hopes that this book will be read by those who have never had to think about the disabled and who will come to see that "there is nothing more significant to be done in a world of such deep injustice than to take the time to be friends with the handicapped." I share his hope and his vision for peace embodied by this book.

David L. Coulter, MD

REFERENCES

American Association on Mental Retardation (2002). *Mental Retardation: Definition, Classification, and Systems of Supports*, 10th Edition. Washington, D.C.: American Association on Mental Retardation.

Coulter, D.L. (2001). Recognition of spirituality in health care: Personal and universal implications. *Journal of Religion, Disability & Health*, 5 (2/3), 1-11.

Coulter, D.L. (2002). The strength of families and individuals. *Journal of Religion, Disability & Health*, 6 (1), 1-5.

Introduction:
Hauerwas on Disability

SUMMARY. Swinton outlines some central aspects of Hauerwas' theology and ethics that relate to the papers in this volume. He clarifies the type of disability that Hauerwas addresses in these papers and draws out the social and political dimensions of Hauerwas' critique. The chapter explores issues of terminology, politics, and citizenship. In so doing this chapter lays down a foundation for the various papers and responses that are presented in the book. *[Article copies available for a fee from The Haworth Document Delivery Service: 1-800-HAWORTH. E-mail address: <docdelivery@haworthpress.com> Website: <http://www.HaworthPress.com> © 2004 by The Haworth Press, Inc. All rights reserved.]*

KEYWORDS. Disability, ethics, theology, liberal society, politics, empowerment

A couple of years ago I had the pleasure of meeting Stanley Hauerwas and spending and afternoon with him. He was in the United Kingdom doing the *Scottish Journal of Theology* lectures at my own university, the University of

John Swinton is Professor in Practical Theology and Pastoral Care, University of Aberdeen, Scotland, UK. Professor Swinton has a background in nursing and hospital chaplaincy and is an ordained minister in the Church of Scotland.

[Haworth co-indexing entry note]: "Introduction: Hauerwas on Disability." Swinton, John. Co-published simultaneously in Journal of Religion, Disability & Health (The Haworth Pastoral Press, an imprint of The Haworth Press, Inc.) Vol. 8, No. 3/4, 2004, pp. 1-9; and: *Critical Reflections on Stanley Hauerwas' Theology of Disability: Disabling Society, Enabling Theology* (ed: John Swinton) The Haworth Pastoral Press, an imprint of The Haworth Press, Inc., 2004, pp. 1-9. Single or multiple copies of this article are available for a fee from The Haworth Document Delivery Service [1-800-HAWORTH, 9:00 a.m. - 5:00 p.m. (EST). E-mail address: docdelivery@haworthpress.com].

Aberdeen in Scotland, United Kingdom. The morning had been interesting to say the least. Stanley had provided an excellent blend of solid, challenging imaginative theology, interspersed with the odd off the cuff comment that caused some of our more conservative students to raise their eyebrows! However, despite the odd bit of controversy the lectures went very well and we were all blessed and challenged.

Midweek I was allocated the task of spending an afternoon entertaining this "strange" visiting Texan professor. Entertaining strangers is not always my greatest gift, but I was happy to oblige. Suffice it to say that any fears I might have had were instantly dismissed as I found myself wrapped up in a fascinating encounter with a man who was warm, deceptively gentle, and fully committed to many of the issues that filled my own life horizons. As we spoke, it became clear that the deep theological and ethical issues that Hauerwas has made a career out of wrestling with were not taken on at a superficial level. There was more to Hauerwas than simply rhetoric and flair. As we talked, I began to develop a picture of a man who understood what it was like to suffer; someone who had experienced the consequences of disability first hand and who knew the practical as well as the theoretical meaning of suffering and joy. As we spent time together it became clear to me that Hauerwas' voice was one which deserved to be listened to, not only by the academic community, but also by the wider community who wrestle with the meaning of being human and living humanly in an age of complexity and change. I left our encounter feeling privileged to have spent time with someone who had taken the time to reflect thoughtfully and critically on the meaning of humanness and who has offered the world some fascinating and challenging insights into what it means for us to live lives which are fully human irrespective of the perceived state of our mental and physical faculties. It is, therefore, with great pleasure that I offer readers the opportunity to share in some of Hauerwas' thinking and to give all of us the opportunity to reflect carefully and thoughtfully on his contribution to our understanding not only of disability, but also of what it means to be human and to live humanly in a complex and rapidly changing world of diversity and change.

ABOUT THIS BOOK

Hauerwas' writings on disability are disparate and diverse. They are to be found in various journal articles and book chapters which have been written over the course of the past thirty years. With one notable exception, there has been no attempt to draw together Hauerwas' thinking on disability (Hauerwas 1986); neither has there been any effort made to reflect critically on the implications of his perspective for the praxis of caring for and offering support to people with disabilities and those who strive to offer such care and support. This volume seeks to address this gap in the continuing process of critical reflection on Hauerwas' work. The book brings together ten of Hauerwas' key essays on disability and draws them into critical dialogue with an international group of practitioners, ethicists, theologians and carers, in an attempt to tease out the significance and contemporary relevance of his contribution to the theology and ethics of developmental disabilities. It concludes with a final new essay from Professor Hauerwas within which he draws together the various threads of reflection and critique and offers some concluding pointers for the future.

The commentators were asked to reflect critically and imaginatively on Hauerwas' work and to draw out that which is relevant and challenging as well as that which is questionable or even mistaken. The result is a rich and fascinating tapestry of thoughts and ideas which clarifies, challenges, enhances, and contextualises Hauerwas' thinking within contemporary theological reflection on disability. It is hoped that the multidisciplinary dialogue presented within this book will enable readers to reflect deeply on Hauerwas' work and to draw out and put into practice that which is relevant for today.

Like all good theologians, Hauerwas' talent lies not simply in what he actually says, but equally in what he challenges others to say. Not everyone agrees with his position and some of the commentators offer some trenchant critiques of his approach and thinking. However, despite their concerns, it is clear that each participant in this book has been challenged by Hauerwas' thinking and forced to work through the issues in new ways. In so doing they have produced some valuable reflections and insights which would not have existed had they not taken the opportunity to engage thoughtfully and constructively with Hauerwas' thinking. For that and much more, I am certain that each person who has contributed to this book feels indebted to Professor Hauerwas. It is our hope that readers will be similarly challenged to move on in their exploration of the true meaning of disability.

The essays and responses presented here were gathered together and edited by Professor Swinton and reflected on by Professor Hauerwas. We hope that they will enable people to see disability differently and in seeing disability differently begin to act differently in the presence of those whom we choose to call 'disabled.'

Hauerwas on Disability

In order to understand the significance of Hauerwas' contribution to the debate about the theology and ethics of disability, it is necessary to begin by doing some basic ground work. It is not possible or necessary here to offer a comprehensive overview of Hauerwas' theology and ethics. This has been done very effectively elsewhere (Berkman and Cartwright 2001; Wells 1998). In the following sections I will outline some of the main points of Hauerwas' general thinking as it relates specifically to the essays presented in this book. The outline is intended to orientate readers within the parameters of Hauerwas' view of the world and to provide them with some initial guidance as to how and why he views disability in the way that he does.

Why Listen to Hauerwas?

It is important to begin by noting the fact that Hauerwas has been advocating for people with disabilities and their families since the late 70s (Hauerwas 1973). To the best of my knowledge no other mainstream theologian has so consistently and trenchantly taken a stand with and for people with developmental disabilities. Whilst some ethicists continue to make the case for the eradication of people with developmental disabilities (Singer 1993), Hauerwas has consistently (if unsystematically) produced a significant critique of practices, attitudes, and philosophical positions which attempt to dehumanise and ultimately eliminate people with intellectual disabilities.

Until relatively recently mainstream theology has not taken the practical and hermeneutical challenge of disability as a serious dimension of theology and praxis. Understandings of disability have traditionally been tied in with ideas of charity, action towards disabled people coming as an end point of a process of ethical reflection on the "poor" or the "weak." Hauerwas has always understood the issues to be much deeper and more profound than simply caring for those whom society perceives as "poor" and "weak." For Hauerwas, the issue at stake is our understanding of the nature of what it means to be human and to live humanly within the coming Kingdom of God. Hauerwas turns the ethic of charity around and begins his ethical reflections with the perspective of a group of people whom society deems to be "poor" and "weak" and as such worthy only of pity and charity. In listening to and taking seriously the experience of people with profound developmental disabilities and their families, Hauerwas offers a response to their challenge which reframes and disturbs our worldviews at both a personal and a socio-political level. Charity is not enough. What is required is a radical change in our perspective. A change which leads us to participate fully in the paradigm shift that was initiated by the life, death, and resurrection of Jesus and which the church has been given responsibility for embodying and living out. It is in wrestling with this process of embodying and living out the gospel that Hauerwas finds genuine revelation in the lives of people with developmental disabilities. But how does Hauerwas come to such a conclusion?

From Charity to Politics:
The Social Construction of Developmental Disabilities

The type of disability that Hauerwas reflects on relates to a group of human beings who are deemed by the majority to have limited communicational skills, restricted or no self care skills, significant intellectual and/or cognitive difficulties and who essentially will have to have some kind of full-time care throughout their lives. Hauerwas uses the term "mental retardation" or "mental handicap" to describe these people. Of course, on reflection, such a description actually raises more questions than it answers: "Whose communication is faulty–carer or cared for?" "Why are *self*-care skills important?" "What makes it difficult for people perceived to have cognitive or intellectual disabilities? The perceived difficulties or the fact that society values highly what they appear not to have?" Nevertheless, this description of people with profound developmental disabilities at least orients us within the general field of human experience that forms the context for Hauerwas' theological and ethical reflections. The important thing to note is that it is not disability in general that is his focus, nor even the whole sweep of developmental disabilities. Rather his focus is on this very particular type of disability or better, this particular way of being human which has become highly problematic within Western liberal societies.

The "Retarded" in Liberal Society

So what is it about this way of being human that so disturbs, fascinates and challenges Hauerwas? Hauerwas has astutely noticed a close and often overlooked connection between the life experiences of people with profound developmental disabilities and the type of society that they find themselves living in. For Hauerwas, post-Enlightenment Western culture is liberal in its worldview, assumptions, and expectations. Liberalism emphasises the importance of reason, rationality, independence, and the capacity for self-advocacy. The assumed norm for authentic human living is that a person should be able to articulate their ideas cognitively, logically, and rationally. From the perspective of liberalism, society is assumed to be an association of free and independent equals. To be a 'person' means that one must be able to live one's life, develop one's potential and develop a purposeful life-course without any necessary reference to others. Importantly, these capacities are not only necessary for entry into the socio-political system, they are also considered necessary for a person to live in a way which can be deemed authentically human (Kittay, pp. 2-4).

The experience of profound developmental disabilities sits uneasily with the expectations, hopes, and dreams of liberal society. In a context within which "clarity of mind and economic productivity determine the value of a human life" (Post 1995, p. 3), people with this type of life experience sit awkwardly on the borders of acceptable humanness. In a "hypercognitive society" (Post 1995, p. 2) within which 'usefulness' and quality of life are judged in accordance with such criteria as independence, rationality, productivity, vitality and fitness, in what sense can those who appear not to have such things be viewed as fully human? How can lives which do not contain such things be called meaningful or purposeful?

This liberal view forms the context for the types of controversies over the nature of personhood which have become so popular, and destructive within medical ethics. For some, the lack of cognitive ability, dependence, and inability to contribute to society inevitably moves people with profound developmental disabilities out of the world of persons and into a strange land of 'in-validity,' within which their personhood is deemed invalid and their stature as full human beings significantly undermined (Swinton 2000; 2001). Such discussions place people with profound developmental disabilities in a very tenuous position, not least because they have no voice in the ongoing discussion. It is in addressing this threat to the humanity of people with developmental disabilities that Hauerwas finds his motivation and drive.

The Community as the "Hermeneutic of the Gospel"

As a counter to the excesses of liberal society, Hauerwas argues for a very particular understanding of the church as a community. He calls for the church to become a community. Such a suggestion is not in itself particularly radical, but this community is of a very particular shape and form. The community of the church is not determined by the epistemology of liberal society. Rather, it is called to be what Lesslie Newbigin has described as "the hermeneutic of the gospel" (Newbigin 1990), that place where the gospel is lived out and interpreted to the world through the actions and character of its participants. "The church is the place where the story of God is enacted, told, and heard" (Hauerwas 1988, p. 101). It is here that the truth about the crucified Jesus is revealed and taught not just through words but in actions and gestures that reveal the nature and truth of the coming peaceable kingdom.

This is an important point. Whereas the church and culture have traditionally assumed truth primarily to be cognitive and propositional, Hauerwas suggests that truth in general and, in particular theological truth, is contextual, to some extent non-cognitive (hence his emphasis on the significance of gesture) and closely bound to particular communities. The church has been profoundly influenced by the worldview and epistemological priorities of liberal culture. Hauerwas calls it back to be what it was intended to be: a community of virtue and character that reveals in its life and actions a radically new vision of humanness and human living based on the life, death, and resurrection of Jesus Christ. Within this community there is 'neither Jew nor Greek, slave nor free, male nor female . . . black nor white, able bodied, and handicapped' (Young 1990, p. 192); here dependence, vulnerability, and weakness are recognised not as deficits, but as a valued fundamental theological truth. As human beings made in the image of God and sustained by grace we are inevitably dependant beings: persons-in-relation (Macmurray 1998). The church is not sustained by intellect or reason but by grace which is manifested in the various gestures of love and revelation which form the fabric of meaningful community.

Hauerwas' vision of community with people with profound developmental disabilities is beautifully illustrated in his reflections on L'Arche in the first essay of this volume, and his subtle but crucial exploration of the tension between propositional truth and truth as it is experienced in community and articulated poetically and profoundly in the work of Jean Vanier. It is within such communities of character that the lie is put to ideas of the necessity of individualism and rationalism for authentic human living. It is within such a community that the humanness and value of people with profound developmental disabilities is recognised and worked out. It is within such a community that we learn to live out the heart of the gospel.

The Problem with Speaking for Disabled People

It could, of course, be argued that Hauerwas is simply using people with developmental disabilities for his own theological ends. This is a criticism that is acknowledged and worked through to some extent by Hauerwas and Bérubé in their reflections in chapter one. However, Hauerwas' dilemma is not unique. Rather, it is a question that we all must bear in mind as we reflect on the lives of people who in some senses are vulnerable, voiceless, and open to abuse and manipulation, albeit implicit and done with good intentions. Having spent a considerable amount of time with Hauerwas' work in putting this volume together, my feeling is that his intentions are genuine and that whilst the danger of manipulating people with disabilities for personal ends remains, his desire remains liberatory and deeply humane. The readers will of course make up their own minds. However, it is probably not insignificant that none of the commentators felt this to be a major issue.

Following on from the line of criticism highlighted above, another accusation that could be levelled at Hauerwas is that he tends to focus on the carers rather than the cared for. The actual voices and lived experiences of people with profound developmental disabilities are not heard loudly in Hauerwas' writings. This may be fair criticism. However, it is criticism that needs to be tempered with the historical contexts of many of the essays. As Linda Treloar points out in her contribution, deinstitutionalization has shifted the locus if not the force of Hauerwas' argument. However, history cannot excuse all things and one is still left wondering why in his most recent essay on disability, written from within a social context where user empowerment and identity politics are firmly on the public agenda, the voice of the person with profound developmental disabilities remains absent. It may be that Hauerwas perceives his primary task as advocating for parents and carers. In itself this is an admirable and crucial task. However, one must still ask the question as to how one can formulate an adequate theological response by listening to and reflecting on only one voice within an ongoing dialogue between carer and cared for.

The Question of Terminology: Who are the "Mentally Retarded?"

Before moving on to explore Hauerwas' thinking in more depth, it is important to be clear just who it is that he is dealing with in the essays presented in this book. Hauerwas' focus is not on disability in general, but on what he describes as "mental retardation" or "mental handicap." These are perhaps unfortunate terms with unpleasant historical connotations. Indeed they become quite problematic for Hauerwas when we take his work into a contemporary context where the history and implications of such terms are much clearer than they would have been when some of the essays were originally written. Limits of space prevent us from exploring the complex issues that surround the continually changing labelling systems which affect the lives of people with perceived cognitive deficits. Some of the responders in this volume touch on these issues, albeit inconclusively. For current purposes it may be suffice to suggest that Hauerwas' use of the term "mental retardation" reflects both the time in which the essays were written and the context from which they came. However, before we criticise Hauerwas too heavily for his use of terminology it is interesting to reflect on the diversity of terminology used by the various responders in this volume. It would appear that the question of names and labels is far from conclusively answered! I would therefore ask readers to take cognisance of the historical and contextual nature of these essays and, as far as possible, not to allow debates over terminology to divert attention from the very important arguments that are worked out in this book.

It will be noted that for the purposes of this introductory essay I have used the term 'developmental disability,' a term which while far from perfect, is currently gaining a degree of acceptability within an international context. However, the debate continues!

CONCLUSION

Despite such concerns, Hauerwas' contribution to the field of disability theology is highly significant. It is my hope that in raising readers' awareness of the potential significance of these essays that the vital issues which emerge will be grasped and worked through and that at the end of the day, all of us will understand more fully the life experience of people with profound developmental disabilities and their families and in so doing, be able to live, love, and care a bit more humanly because of that.

REFERENCES

Hauerwas, Stanley. (1988). *Christian Existence Today: Essays on Church, World, and Living in Between.* The Labyrinth Press, Durham, North Carolina.

_____(1973). 'Christian Care of the Retarded.' *Theology Today July.* Vol. 30-2, pp. 130-137.

Kittay, Eva Feder. *Love's Labor: Essays on Women, Equality, and Dependency.* Routledge. 1998.

Macmurray, John. (1998). *Persons in Relation.* Humanity Books.

Newbigin, Lesslie. (1990). *The Gospel in a Pluralist Society.* Grand Rapids: Wm. B. Eerdmans Publishing Co.

Post, Stephen. (1995). *The Moral Challenge of Alzheimer's Disease.* London: Johns Hopkins Press.

Swinton, John. (2000). *Resurrecting the Person: Friendship and the Care of People with Mental Health Problems.* Nashville: Abingdon.

_____*Spirituality and mental health care: Rediscovering a "forgotten" dimension.* (2001a). London: Jessica Kingsley Publishers.

_____ (2001b). *A space to listen: The spiritual care of people with learning disabilities.* London: Mental Health Foundation.

Young, F. *Face to Face: A narrative essay in the theology of suffering.* T & T Clark, Edinburgh 1990, p. 192.

Chapter 1

Timeful Friends:
Living with the Handicapped

Stanley Hauerwas, PhD

[From *Sanctify Them in the Truth: Holiness Exemplified*. Nashville: Abingdon Press, 1999, pp. 143-156]. (Also published by Continuum International Publishing Group, T & T Clark)]. Reprinted with permission.

SUMMARY. In this paper Hauerwas reflects on the significance of the L'Arche communities as exemplars of the true nature of Christian community. He explores the philosophy and theology of Jean Vanier as a mode of embodied theology. Hauerwas reflects critically on Michael Bérubé's book *Life as We Know It*, in which he describes his experiences

---

The author would like to acknowledge Brett Webb-Mitchell's account of Vanier as well as his study of L'Arche: *L'Arche: An Ethnographic Study of Persons with Disabilities Living in a Community with Non-Disabled People*, PhD Dissertation: University of North Carolina, 1988. Webb-Mitchell has published a series of books that explore the theological significance of the mentally handicapped and, in particular, how friendship with the handicapped is possible. See his *God Plays Piano, too* (New York: Crossroads, 1993), *Unexpected Guests at God's Banquet* (New York: Crossroads, 1994), and *Dancing with Disabilities* (Cleveland: United Church Press, 1996).

[Haworth co-indexing entry note]: "Timeful Friends: Living with the Handicapped." Hauerwas, Stanley. Co-published simultaneously in *Journal of Religion, Disability & Health* (The Haworth Pastoral Press, an imprint of The Haworth Press, Inc.) Vol. 8, No. 3/4, 2004, pp. 11-25; and: *Critical Reflections on Stanley Hauerwas' Theology of Disability: Disabling Society, Enabling Theology* (ed: John Swinton) The Haworth Pastoral Press, an imprint of The Haworth Press, Inc., 2004, pp. 11-25. Single or multiple copies of this article are available for a fee from The Haworth Document Delivery Service [1-800-HAWORTH, 9:00 a.m. - 5:00 p.m. (EST). E-mail address: docdelivery@haworthpress.com].

http://www.haworthpress.com/web/JRDH
Digital Object Identifier: 10.1300/J095v8n03_02

with his son who has Down's syndrome. In drawing together the perspectives of Bérubé and Vanier, Hauerwas explores the nature of disability in liberal society and presents an ethical and moral perspective which calls us to take seriously the significance of meaningful community marked by friendship and 'timefullness.' Such a community will enable us to become 'friends of time,' a form of friendship which seeks meaningful ways to 'be with' and not to 'do for' people with developmental disabilities.

KEYWORDS. L'Arche, Vanier, wisdom, friendship, community, ethics

L'Arche is special, in the sense that we are trying to live in community with people who are mentally handicapped. Certainly we want to help them grow and reach the greatest independence possible. But before "doing for them," we want to "be with them." The particular suffering of the person who is mentally handicapped, as of all marginal people, is a feeling of being excluded, worthless, and unloved. It is through everyday life in community and the love that must be incarnate in this, that handicapped people can begin to discover that they have a value, that they are loved and so lovable. (Vanier 1979, p. 3)

Individual growth towards love and wisdom is slow. A community's growth is even slower. Members of a community have to be friends of time. They have to learn that many things will resolve themselves if they are given enough time. It can be a great mistake to want, in the name of clarity and truth, to push things too quickly to a resolution. Some people enjoy confrontation and highlighting divisions. This is not always healthy. It is better to be a friend of time. But clearly too, people should not pretend that problems don't exist by refusing to listen to the rumblings of discontent; they must be aware of the tensions. (Vanier 1977, p. 80)

Our focal point of fidelity at L'Arche is to live with handicapped people in the spirit of the Gospel and the Beatitudes. "To live with" is different from "to do for." It doesn't simply mean eating at the same table and sleeping under the same roof. It means that we create relationships of gratuity, truth and interdependence, that we listen to the handicapped people; that we recognize and marvel at their gifts. The day we become no more than professional workers and educational therapists is the day we stop being L'Arche–although of course "living with" does not exclude this professional aspect. (Vanier 1979, p. 106)

ON THE ETHICS OF WRITING
ABOUT THE ETHICS OF THE CARE
OF THE MENTALLY HANDICAPPED

Every time I write about the mentally handicapped I make a promise to myself that it will be the last time I write about this subject. Yet here I am breaking my promise once again. I published my first essay on the mentally handicapped over twenty years ago. I have continued to speak and write about the mentally handicapped ever since. Surely, one would think, by now I have said all I have to say. Of course, such an attitude, that is, that I have said what I have to say, is that of an intellectual. People who really care about the mentally handicapped never run out of things to say, since they do not write "about" the mentally handicapped precisely because they do not view the mentally handicapped as just another "subject." They write for and, in some sense, with the mentally handicapped. To be able to write for and with the mentally handicapped requires that you know people who are mentally handicapped. By "know" I mean you must be *with* the handicapped in a way they may be able to claim you as a friend. I was once so claimed, but over the last few years I have not enjoyed such a friendship. So, when I now write about the ethics of caring for the mentally handicapped, I fear I am not talking about actual people but more of my memories of the mentally handicapped. When they become an abstraction, moreover, we can begin to think we must provide "reasons" for their existence or, worse, discover meaning in why we care for them.

Jean Vanier, as the passages at the beginning of this essay make clear, feels no need to find meaning in why L'Arche homes exist. I call attention to the tension I feel in yet once again writing about the mentally handicapped, because my difficulty illustrates the challenge facing all who care for them. How do we care for the mentally handicapped without allowing the reasons we are tempted to give for such care to distort what should be our relation to those for whom we care? To make the question even more difficult–"How do we care for the mentally handicapped in such a manner which would forestall our felt need to provide reasons why we should care for the mentally handicapped, thereby rendering their lives unintelligible?" After all, both the existence and care of those of us who are considered "normal" is not thought to require justification. Why is the existence and/or care of the "mentally handicapped" singled out as presenting a special problem?

In truth my difficulty with writing about the mentally handicapped did not begin with my isolation from the handicapped. From the beginning I have always felt a bit duplicitous when I addressed the subject of the mentally handicapped and their care. In fact, I have not ever really written about the mentally handicapped. No matter how much I care for the mentally handicapped, I have been haunted by the presumption that my "interest" in them and my writing about them has been part of an intellectual agenda that makes them useful to me. Once I had been drawn into the world of the mentally handicapped, however, it did not take me long to realize they were the crack I desperately needed to give concreteness to my critique of modernity. No group exposes the pretensions of the humanism that shapes the practices of modernity more thoroughly than the mentally handicapped. Our humanism entails we care for them once they are among us, once we are stuck with them; but the same humanism cannot help but think that, all things considered, it would be better if they did not exist. As modern people we think we are meant to be autonomous beings.

In view of such an overpowering presumption, how do we make sense of those among us whose very existence can be nothing but dependence? We live in cultures for which rationality and consciousness are taken to be the very essence of what makes us human. What are we to make of those who will never, even with the best efforts, be able to read or write? Should they be considered human? Examples of how the mentally handicapped render problematic some of the most cherished conceits of modernity are legion. For example, in his *Life as We Know It: A Father, a Family, and an Exceptional Child*, Michael Bérubé tells of the birth and care he and his wife have given to their Down's Syndrome son, Jamie (Bérubé 1996). His is a wonderful story of how two college professors found their lives reshaped by their son's disability. I have nothing but admiration for the way they have accepted and cared for their son. The story Bérubé tells of their struggle to keep Jamie alive and to secure appropriate medical care is at once as inspiring as it is humane. Moreover, Professor Bérubé has read his Foucault. He knows that some of the most humane forms of "treatment" may be but forms of control. He even knows that the most humane accounts of justice in modernity, such as those of Rawls and Habermas, cannot help his son.

That such accounts of justice require that we shed our individual idiosyncrasies make the existence of his son irresolvably problematic. As Bérubé puts it,

> There isn't a chance in the world that James Lyon Bérubé could come to the table independently of "interests," independent of cognitive and social idiosyncrasies legible to all, independent of either a genetic makeup

or a social apparatus that constructs him as "abnormal." The society that fosters Jamie's independence must start from an understanding of his dependencies, and any viable conception of justice has to take the concrete bodies and "private," idiosyncratic interest of individuals like Jamie into account, or it will be of no account at all. (Bérubé 1996, p. 248)

Bérubé may not appreciate the considerable differences between the accounts of justice by Rawls and Habermas but I think he rightly intuits that such differences in the face of the mentally handicapped do not amount to much. Bérubé criticizes Rawls and Habermas for succumbing to "a curious Enlightenment fantasy, the idea that once we boil away all the idiosyncrasies and impurities of the irrational human race, we can come up with some perfectly neutral, rational, disinterested character who can play the language-game of justice as if it were a contest in which he or she had no stake" (Bérubé 1996, p. 247).

Yet Bérubé's criticism of Rawls and Habermas rings hollow in the light of his own narrative. He either cannot or does not choose to make intelligible his admirable commitment to Jamie. For example, with great candor Bérubé tells us that he and his wife are as pro-choice after the birth of Jamie as they were prior to his birth. Indeed, he notes that they intentionally did not use amniocentesis, assuming they would "just love the baby all the more" if the baby was born with Down Syndrome. He confesses such a stance was "blithe and uninformed" and that if they had known that their child's life "would be suffering and misery for all concerned" they might have chosen to have an abortion (Bérubé 1996, p. 47). Bérubé notes, however, that it is extremely difficult to discuss Jamie in this way. Just as it was hard to talk about him as a medicalized being when he was in the ICU, it is still harder to "talk about him in terms of our philosophical beliefs about abortion and prenatal testing. That's partly because these issues are so famously divisive and emotionally charged, but it's also because we can no longer frame any such questions about our child now that he's here" (Bérubé 1996, p. 48).

"Now that he is here" is the nub of the matter. Bérubé does not pretend to be able to do more than represent Jamie "now that he is here." Indeed, he takes that as his ethical and aesthetic task–to help us to imagine Jamie and to imagine what he might think of our ability to imagine him. Just as the Bérubé's look forward to the day that Jamie will be able to eat at the "big" table, to feed himself tacos, burgers, and pizza, to set the table even if such a setting is somewhat "random," so Bérubé's job:

> is to represent my son, to set his place at our collective table. But I know I am merely trying my best to prepare for the day he sets his own place. For I have no sweeter dream than to imagine–aesthetically and ethically

and parentally–that Jamie will someday be his own advocate, his own author, his own best representative." (Bérubé 1996, p. 264)

How sad. All Bérubé can imagine for Jamie is that he be "his own author." That Bérubé can imagine no other future is not his fault. His imagination reflects the same limits that formed the conceptions of justice he found so unsatisfactory. What other possibility could there be in a world in which God does not exist? What other politics is available for those like the Bérubé's when the church has been reduced to reinforcing the sentimentalities of contemporary humanism? Bérubé has been gifted with Jamie, but he lacks the practices of a community that would provide the resources for narrating his own and Jamie's life.

That is the "crack" I have exploited in the interest of a theological agenda. In short I have used the "now that he is here" as a resource to illumine Christian speech. As Christians we know we have not been created to be "our own authors," to be autonomous. We are creatures. Dependency, not autonomy, is one of the ontological characteristics of our lives. That we are creatures, moreover, is but a reminder that we are created for and with one another. We are not just accidentally communal, but we are such by necessity. We were not created to be alone. We cannot help but desire and delight in the reality of the other, even the other born with a difference we call mentally handicapped. Our dependency, our need for one another, means that we will suffer as well as know joy. Our incompleteness at once makes possible the gifts that make life possible as well as the unavoidability of suffering. Such suffering, moreover, may seem pointless (see Hauerwas 1990 for a further development of this point). Yet, at least for Christians, such suffering should not tempt us to think our task is to eliminate those whose suffering seems pointless. Christians are, or at least should be, imbedded in a narrative that makes possible a sharing of lives with one another that enables us to go on in the face of the inexplicable. For Christians the mentally handicapped do not present a peculiar challenge. That the mentally handicapped are constituted by narratives they have not chosen simply reveals the character of our lives. That some people are born with a condition that we have come to label as being mentally handicapped does not indicate a fundamental difference between them and the fact that we must all be born. The question is not whether we can justify the mentally handicapped, but whether we live any longer in a world that can make sense of having children. At the very least, Christians believe that our lives are constituted by the hope we have learned through Christ's cross and resurrection that makes morally intelligible the bringing of children into a world as dark as our own.

I have not made these arguments to try to convince people constituted by the narratives of modernity that they should believe in God. Such an argument could not help but make God a deus ex machina, which not only demeans God, but God's creation as well. Rather, my concern is to help Christians locate those practices that help us understand better why our willingness to welcome the mentally handicapped should not be surprising given the triune nature of the God we worship. In other words, I have used the mentally handicapped as material markers necessary to show that Christian speech can and in fact does make claims about the way things are. Theologically, thinking about the mentally handicapped helps us see, moreover, that claims about the way things are cannot be separated from the way we should live. By subjecting the mentally handicapped to this agenda, one might object, am I not also exemplifying the desperate attempt I have criticized in others to find some "meaning" in the existence and care of the handicapped? I would obviously like to answer with a quick denial, but as I indicated above, the question rightly continues to haunt me. That it does so, I think, is partly because I am not sure how one rightly responds to such a challenge.

What sense are we to make of the care given to the mentally handicapped in a world of limited resources? I think the answer requires the reshaping of the question–a reshaping, I believe, gestured at in the work of people like Jean Vanier. For we will only know why we do what we do by the exemplary lives of those like Vanier who teach us how to live with those we call the mentally handicapped. So I can do no better than to turn our attention to his work.

On "Using" the Mentally Handicapped

Before I turn to Vanier, however, I want to expose a narrative that I suspect may inform and shape questions about the "use" of the mentally handicapped–that is, the kind of problematic that has shaped what I have just said about my own disease with my use of the mentally handicapped. It is, moreover, a narrative that I think is particularly pernicious, not only for the care of the mentally handicapped, but for any human relations, including our relations to animals and nature. This narrative received its most eloquent expression as well as its most adequate defence in the second formulation of Kant's categorical imperative–"Act so that you treat humanity, whether in your own person or in that of another, always as an end and never as a means only" (Kant 1959, p. 47). For many, such an imperative seems to embody our highest ideal. Kant certainly did not think of it as an ideal, but rather thought such an imperative constitutive of any moral act that deserves the description, "moral." Unfortunately this results in the creation of the realm of "morality" that moderns assume can be distinguished from economics, politics, or, more importantly, manners. Once such a realm exists, some people then think they have to think about the "ethics" of the care of the retarded.

The power of this narrative–that is, that we should treat one another as ends and not means, is revealed for modern people by the very fact that we cannot imagine anyone seriously challenging it as a statement of what we should at least always try to do. One may doubt the existence of God, but it seems everyone agrees with the ideal that we ought never to treat one another simply as a means. The way we often put the matter is that every human being should be treated with dignity. Of course, like most abstractions, it is very hard to know what it means to treat others as ends. That most human relations require we treat one another as means does not seem to call into question the assumption that we ought not so to do. Whatever the difficulty may be in concrete specification of treating another as an end, we continue to think we all would prefer to be treated as an end, not a means This seems particularly to be the case when it comes to the mentally handicapped. We presume that the improvement in the care of the mentally handicapped over this century derives from our commitment to treat them as persons deserving respect–that is, as ends in themselves.

There is, of course, the troubling problem of whether the mentally handicapped possess the characteristics necessary to be counted as persons. If they do not, for example, possess minimal forms of rationality, can they be considered persons deserving of respect? Is the care of such beings then to be considered supererogatory? Such questions may be considered too theoretical to be of interest, but if resources become scarce, questions about the care of the mentally handicapped can begin to have frightening implications.

The language of means and ends often has peculiar power in the treatment the mentally handicapped actually receive. The ethic that often shapes critiques of institutionalization of the handicapped, that creates the demand for their normalization, that requires they receive appropriate medical treatment, is one that assumes they too should be treated as ends not as "means only." (It is important to note that Kant quite sensibly assumed that it is sometimes permissible to treat people as means. What the imperative excludes is that treatment as a means occludes their status as ends. Of course this but creates the problem of how we are to know when someone has ever been treated as a "means only.") That any restrictions on the mentally handicapped should be the "least restrictive" seems to require that the mentally handicapped are to be treated as far as possible like anyone else. Yet what "as far as possible" means is not easily determined.

For example, Michael Bérubé observes how the Foucauldian question haunts the humanities:

> Is it wrong to *speak for* others, to assume that one can represent the interests of another in a faithful and transparent way? How can one be an advocate for the mentally retarded while believing that institutions never

die and that every act of representation is also an act of usurpation? Is there no way to have faith in Camelot, in Special Olympics, in Advocacy? (Bérubé 1996, p. 112)

Bérubé answers that whatever he may believe about the history of madness, sexuality, incarceration, it is impossible to act as a Foucauldian when it comes to Jamie.

> We *have* to act, for both theoretical and practical reasons, in the belief that these agencies can benefit our child, even as the sorry history of institutionalization weighs on our brains like a nightmare. To act in any other way, to indict all such institutions across the board, would be to consign Jamie to the kind of self-fulfilling prophecy that follows from unearned cynicism: *We know they can't help, so why bother?* It would be hard to imagine a more irresponsible attitude toward his life's prospects. (Bérubé 1996, p. 113)

Yet Bérubé knows, as every parent of the mentally handicapped knows, that they are caught in what seems an irresolvable conundrum. In order for your child to receive appropriate care they must be labelled–retarded, handicapped, Down syndrome–but the labels can become self-fulfilling prophecies; or worse, the labels can legitimate the intervention of others into their children's lives that often only benefits the agents of intervention.

This becomes particularly troubling when the agent of intervention is an institution called the state. Parents want their child treated as an end, with respect, but in a social ethos dominated by an ethic of respect, their children can only be treated as a means. Which I think brings us back to Kant and why the second formulation of the categorical imperative is not only inadequate to help us understand the place of the mentally handicapped but for any account of morality. For what is often forgotten is that Kant's formulation of the categorical imperative presupposes an account of existence that is without ultimate telos. What purpose there is results from human freedom now understood as an end in itself. Humanity is forced to impose meaning on a mechanistic world whose only meaning is to be found in our existence as humans. Human behavior is subject to mechanistic explanation as any part of nature. We remain ends only to the extent we can will ourselves to be such. What such a view of the world cannot do is to allow us to ask "What are people for?" (Berry 1990). Such a question presupposes that creation, all that is, has a purpose that is not a function of our self-generating will. On such a view human beings have a telos that allows a distinction to be drawn between man-as-he-happens-to-be and man-as-he-could-be-if-he-realized-his-essential-nature.

Ethics is the science that is to enable men to understand how they make the transition from the former state to the latter (MacIntyre 1984, p. 52). Such a transition, moreover, requires a community, and the purpose of the community for which we are created is nothing less than friendship with one another. From such a perspective we can begin to appreciate how few resources the means/ends manner of thinking provides for helping us understand the care of the mentally handicapped. Of course, we "use" the mentally handicapped, but we are here to be of use to one another. The notion that any use we make of one another can only be justified if it is done voluntarily can now be seen as one of the peculiar sentimentalities of modernity that results in self-supervision all the more tyrannical since what we do is allegedly what we want to do. That the mentally handicapped are subject to care for their own good–a good they may not have chosen–is not an indication that such care is misguided, but rather requires that the good that such care is serving be properly named. After all, they (like us who are not retarded) exist to serve and to be served for our mutual upbuilding. As Christians we should not feel embarrassed to discover that the mentally handicapped among us help us better understand the narrative that constitutes the very purpose of our existence. That such is the case does not "justify" their existence, but then their existence no more than our existence from a Christian perspective requires justification. We are free to help them just to the extent we no longer feel the necessity to justify their existence. The form such "help" takes can only be discovered relative to the tasks of the community necessary to sustain the practices for the discovery and care of the goods held in common. Put in terms I used above, Christians do not use the mentally handicapped as an affront to a world without purpose, but we should not be surprised that the Christian refusal to abandon the mentally handicapped to such a world will be seen as an affront.

We must confess as Christians, however, that our care of the mentally handicapped has been shaped more by the means/end narrative than by that of Christ. As a result, in the name of care we too often subject the handicapped to therapies based on mechanistic presumptions that promise "results" rather than community. That is why the alternative Vanier represents is so important. For L'Arche offers an imaginative portrayal of what a purposive community might look like in which the mentally handicapped serve and are served. Put metaphysically, the practices that constitute L'Arche rightly assume that being is prior to knowing. Questions about what "meaning" the mentally handicapped may or may not have are questions shaped by habits that assume the priority of epistemological questions. Bérubé's "now that he is here," reveals that the priorities of being cannot be repressed.

Vanier's Wisdom

I am aware, of course, that I will be accused of romanticizing Vanier and the L'Arche movement. Yet as Vanier reminds us,

> Too many communities are founded on dreams and fine words; there is much talk about love, truth, and peace. Marginal people are demanding. Their cries are cries of truth because they sense the emptiness of many of our words; they can see the gap between what we say and what we live. (Vanier 1979, p. 200)

No community can be self-correcting in principle. Criticism is possible only when there are those present who constitute a critical edge. Vanier, whose own presence for L'Arche creates a problem just to the extent some may think L'Arche depends on him, is surely right to suggest that communities like L'Arche at least have some purchase of being truthful to the extent they understand that truth often is spoken by those who cannot speak. Such communities are by necessity constituted by the practice of hospitality. This is not always easy, given Vanier's understanding of community as a grouping of people "who have left their own milieu to live with others under the same roof, and work from a new vision of human beings and their relationships with each other and with God" (Vanier 1979, p. 2). Such communities can easily become ingrown and protective, but for a community that has learned to live with the handicapped such protectiveness can only be destructive. The crucial question is not whether people are to be welcomed, but who is to make the decision who is to be welcomed and how. According to Vanier, in L'Arche communities those best able to discern who should be welcomed are the handicapped. "They have been in the community for a long time, often for longer than the assistants, and sometimes longer than the person in charge. It is important to consult these handicapped people before we welcome someone in distress" (Vanier 1979, p. 197).

I am never sure how to characterize Vanier's observations about L'Arche. It seems right, however, that most of what he has to tell us takes the form of aphorisms–that is, short bursts of hard won wisdom not easily systemized or brought to a point. Wisdom is constituted by judgements about matters that matter. Yet to be wise requires we be part of traditions that form people like Vanier who can say what we all might see or experience, but lack the ability to say what we see. In short, if Vanier had not spent years living with the mentally handicapped he would not have acquired the skills to now speak with and for the handicapped.

The wisdom that he shares with us, gentle though it be, cannot help but disrupt our lives. We read Vanier because we want to know how to do, if not be, good; but in knowing how to do good, we also discover that the subject is not the mentally handicapped, but us. For the great shock for many of us who want to be of help to the handicapped because we think they are weak, is to discover our own weakness. As Vanier observes,

> It is always easier to accept the weakness of handicapped people–we are there precisely because we expect it–than our own weakness that often takes us by surprise! We want to see only good qualities in ourselves and other assistants. Growth begins when we start to accept our own weakness. (Vanier 1979, p. 88)

What, moreover, could be more threatening for the handicapped than for them to expose our own sense of helplessness and loneliness? To be able to be with the mentally handicapped without being "helpful" is what L'Arche is about. It is slow work. Indeed, to be capable of such work means, as Vanier puts it, we have "to be great friends of time" (Vanier 1979, p. 80). We have to become not only friends of time, but friends of those who make such time possible. And to make such time possible is to call upon One who, though outside of time, has entered into our time to be with us and to befriend us. We have to learn how to receive the friendship the mentally handicapped offer to us.

When friendship encourages fidelity, it is the most beautiful thing of all. Aristotle calls it the flower of virtue; it has the gratuity of the flower. On the dark days, we need the refuge of friendship. When we feel flat or fed up, a letter from a friend can bring back peace and confidence. The Holy Spirit uses small things to comfort and strengthen us (Vanier 1979, p. 135).

Our care of the mentally handicapped and their care of us is in the small things we do for one another. "Community is made of the gentle concern that people show each other every day. It is made of small gestures, of services and sacrifices which say 'I love you' and 'I'm happy to be with you' " (Vanier 1979, p. 26). Vanier confesses that when he feels tired he goes to La Forestiere. La Forestiere is a house in his community where none of the nine or so people who live there can talk and most cannot walk. They must express their hearts and emotions through their bodies. The assistants at La Forestiere cannot work at their rhythm, but at that of the handicapped.

Things have to go at a pace which can welcome their least expression; because they have no verbal skills, they have no way of enforcing their views by raising their voice. So the assistants have to be the more attentive to the many non-verbal communications, and this adds greatly to their ability to welcome the whole person. They become increasingly people of welcome and compassion. The slower rhythm and even the presence of the handicapped people makes me slow down, switch off my efficiency motor, rest and recognize the presence of God. The poorest people have an extraordinary power to heal the wounds in our hearts if we welcome them, they nourish us (Vanier 1979, pp. 139-40).

We, that is those of us external to the world of L'Arche communities, are tempted to characterize their work in heroic terms. But that is not how they understand what they do. As Vanier observes, love does not mean doing extraordinary things, but rather knowing how to do ordinary things with tenderness. He calls our attention to the significance of Jesus' "hidden life"–the thirty years he spent in Nazareth when no one knew he was son of God. He lived family and community life in humility working with wood and having his life constituted by the small happenings of such a village. Jesus' hidden life is the model for all community life (Vanier 1979, p. 220). In his life we are given the time to be friends of the timeful friends we call the mentally handicapped.

Doing Things with Vanier

To call attention to Vanier's witness is dangerous just to the extent it is so powerful. He and his friends' presence is too strong for most of us. We cannot imagine reproducing his work in our lives. It requires too much time, it requires too much "labor intensive involvement," it requires people willing to have their lives turned inside out, it assumes that what Christians believe about the world is true and can be lived. For many such requirements and assumptions seem utopian.

Yet they cannot be utopian because L'Arche communities exist. No doubt those in L'Arche often are less than they would wish, but that such a wish forms their desires indicates that they do not think they are pursuing some unrealizable ideal. Moreover, their witness remains crucial for the rest of us are not part of their community; for without such examples imaginations lack the resources to know that what we have become used to doing is not done by necessity. Without L'Arche, anything I or any other theologian might have to say could not help but be empty. L'Arche literally gives weight, gives body, of the world we Christians know as Gospel.

Because Vanier and his friends are so embodied by and in the story of Christ, they feel no need to give meaning to the lives of the mentally handicapped. They feel no need to justify the care they give to the mentally handicapped. They do not think they need to justify their "use" of the mentally handicapped. Such questions and problems do not arise because you do not need to ask such questions about your friends. Friends need no justification. Friendship is a gift and, like most significant gifts, it is surrounded by mystery. We finally cannot explain friendship anymore than we can explain our existence. We can only delight in our friends. Without such delight our care of the mentally handicapped cannot help but seem pointless. Without delight the professional skills we gain to try to help the mentally handicapped can quickly become part of a mechanistic world of control. Vanier and his friends are certainly not disdainful of the wonderful technologies that have been developed to help the handicapped (Vanier 1979, p. 106). Rather they see that such technologies can too easily become ends in themselves no longer serving friendship.

Yet, is all this finally just "too Christian?" Vanier, after all, is obviously a person shaped by Catholic practice and thought. Vanier observes:

> As I think of all the communities throughout the world, struggling for growth, yearning to answer the call of Jesus and of the poor, I realize the need for a universal shepherd, a shepherd who yearns for unity, who has clarity of vision, who calls forth communities and who holds all people. I was deeply touched by the election of John-Paul I and even more touched by the election of John-Paul II. How long will it take before people realize this deep need? How long will it take for Catholics to understand the depths of their gifts and to be confounded in humility? How long will it take Catholics to recognize the beauty and gift in the Protestant churches, especially their love of Scripture and of announcing the Word? And one day will Protestant churches discover the immensity of riches hidden in the Eucharist? Yes, I yearn for this day. (Vanier 1979, p. 104)

How can what is learned in L'Arche be possible in a secular and pluralist world? I do not know for sure how Vanier would answer, but I suspect his answer might be something like this. What is possible in L'Arche is possible anywhere we find people willing to learn to live with the mentally handicapped. After all, the God that is celebrated in L'Arche is God. Such a God knows no boundaries. If such a God can make the mentally handicapped claim some of us as friends, surely such a God will be found among those who know not God. That such is the case after all is why what Christians believe about the world is called "good news." For is it not wonderful to discover in a world as terrible as this that God has created the time, given us friends of time in time, so that we might learn to be friends with one another and, yes, even God?

REFERENCES

Berry, Wendell. (1990) *What Are People For?* San Francisco: North Point Press.
Bérubé, Michael. (1996) *Life As We Know It: A Father, a Family, and an Exceptional Child.* New York: Pantheon Books.

Hauerwas, Stanley. (1990) *Naming the Silences: God, Medicine, and the Problem of Suffering*. Grand Rapids: Eerdmans.

Kant, Immanuel. (1959) *Foundations of the Metaphysics of Morals*. Translated by Lewis White Beck. New York: Liberal Arts Press.

Vanier, Jean. (1979) *Community and Growth*. London: Darton, Longman, and Todd.

Response:
The Need of Strangers

Jean Vanier

SUMMARY. In this paper Jean Vanier responds to Hauerwas' essay by exploring the nature of humanness. Drawing on the thinking of Michael Ignatieff he examines the essence of human need, presenting a case for the centrality of love and respect for human flourishing. People need to have their basic needs fulfilled, but if their deeper needs for love and respect are not met, the possibility of happiness and fulfillment is limited if not impossible. For many people with developmental disabilities it is lack of love and respect which hinders them most in their search for fulfillment. He argues that living in L'Arche is a way of life and an 'attitude towards life' within which these deeper needs are viewed as central for all people, an attitude which is embodied in L'Arche's way of life *with* people who have disabilities. The question is, how might we go about creating a society where there is more love? *[Article copies available for a fee from The Haworth Document Delivery Service: 1-800-HAWORTH. E-mail address: <docdelivery@haworthpress.com> Website: <http://www.HaworthPress.com> © 2004 by The Haworth Press, Inc. All rights reserved.]*

KEYWORDS. Human need, love, respect, community, humanness

Jean Vanier is the founder of L'Arche, an international network of communities for people with disabilities. He lives in L'Arche in Trosly-Breuil where L'Arche was founded in 1964.

[Haworth co-indexing entry note]: "Response: The Need of Strangers." Vanier, Jean. Co-published simultaneously in *Journal of Religion, Disability & Health* (The Haworth Pastoral Press, an imprint of The Haworth Press, Inc.) Vol. 8, No. 3/4, 2004, pp. 27-30; and: *Critical Reflections on Stanley Hauerwas' Theology of Disability: Disabling Society, Enabling Theology* (ed: John Swinton) The Haworth Pastoral Press, an imprint of The Haworth Press, Inc., 2004, pp. 27-30. Single or multiple copies of this article are available for a fee from The Haworth Document Delivery Service [1-800-HAWORTH, 9:00 a.m. - 5:00 p.m. (EST). E-mail address: docdelivery@haworthpress.com].

http://www.haworthpress.com/web/JRDH
© 2004 by The Haworth Press, Inc. All rights reserved.
Digital Object Identifier: 10.1300/J095v8n03_03

The more I continue on my journey with men and women with disabilities, particularly with intellectual disabilities, the more I realize that what we are living together in L'Arche is for all people and touches the fundamental question of the relationship between strength and weakness.

In his book, *The Need of Strangers*, Michael Ignatieff distinguishes between fundamental or basic human needs which, if they are attended to, permit people to live or to survive, from those needs which, if attended to, permit people to flourish, to grow and to attain human maturity (Ignatieff 1989, p. 10). The first are food, lodging, education, medical help, etc. The second are love, respect, dignity, and friendship. The first can be legislated for, the second cannot. If one can order someone not to steal or abuse the property or person of another, one cannot order someone to love. A doctor must prescribe the right medicine for a patient but nobody can oblige him to meet the patient and prescribe the medicine with kindness and respect for the patient.

The need to be loved, appreciated, and treated with respect is of course a universal need. It is at the heart of our attitudes in L'Arche towards people with disabilities. It is–or at least should be–the same attitude towards those who are called to be assistants in L'Arche or board members, neighbours, all people whether or not they come from the same culture or religious tradition as us. In order for them to grow to greater maturity, they too need to be loved and treated with respect.

How then do we learn to treat with respect people who despise and reject those who have an intellectual disability? They are like enemies to such people and so become our enemy. The same can be said of assistants in L'Arche or board members who are caught up in power struggles and the desire to prove that their ideas and ways of doing things are the best. The same can actually be said of people with disabilities who do not want to be loved and appreciated, who are so convinced that they are awful that they act in such a way to prove that they are awful.

This of course touches the whole question of maturity. What does it mean to become a mature human person, to become whole? I can see the value of normalisation and reinsertion but I find that such ideas are too limited. I have seen people with disabilities who make enough money to live alone in an apartment and who close themselves up in their own world, with fast foods and television. They are perhaps normal according to the ways of society, but are they happy and fulfilled in such circumstances? Are they able to attain the maturity they could have if they were not closed up in an ideal of normalisation and reinsertion?

This brings me back to the basic question Stanley Hauerwas wrestles with: *what does it mean to be human?* My own experience and I imagine the experience of many, is that some people appear to be fulfilled and happy while others are angry, fearful, and closed in on themselves. What helps people to move out from themselves to another or others? People move towards others if their basic needs and their deeper needs are fulfilled. People can grow to happiness, to openness and to human fulfillment according to their possibilities if they have friends who truly love and respect them; friends who are kind to them.

Living in L'Arche is a way of life, an attitude towards life. It implies a philosophy and an anthropology. The life lived in L'Arche challenges us to reflect deeply on what it means to be human. The fruit of such reflection enables us to recognise the simple fact that to be human is to help others to attain maturity and human fulfillment.

WHAT IS HUMAN FULFILLMENT?

Experience has shown me that fulfillment is not only found in the acquisition of knowledge, power, success, reputation, and wealth. It is instead discovered primarily in our capacity to love others, to be compassionate to those who are weak, to cooperate with others, to be open to new ideas and to people who are different. Human fulfillment is realised in the way we use our capacities and our knowledge for other peoples' growth. No one is an island. We are all called to love, be it in family, with friends, as part of a town or neighbourhood. We need each other, especially when we are sick or in anguish. We are all parts of a much wider world.

When we begin to think in this way it becomes clear that people with intellectual disabilities are leading us into much larger questions: How might we help assistants grow to greater love and find greater human fulfillment? How can each person be helped to grow into that maturity? Can a society be truly human, a place of justice and peace, if we are not all–or at least the majority of the people–growing towards that fulfillment of love?

What has struck me is how people with disabilities, as "different" as they may be, have a secret power to touch and open other people's hearts. Many young and less young people come to L'Arche without any experience with people who are weak; they come "to help," but they soon discover that in fact they are being helped! Their hearts and minds are being opened. They discover how prejudiced they were. They realise that they do not have to become money-makers or success seekers. There is another way of being and of living, another meaning to life different to what they hear in the media and even in school or at university.

Is it possible that people who are the most rejected and pushed down are the ones who can teach us what it means to be human and lead us to peace? Let me quote from *Expecting Adam* by Martha Beck:

> This is the story of two Harvard driven academics who found out in the mid-pregnancy that their unborn son would be retarded. They decided to allow their baby to be born. What they did not realize is that they themselves were the ones who would be "born," infants in a new world where Harvard professors are the slow learners and retarded babies are the master teachers. (Beck 2000, p. 7)

What is true for people with disabilities is true for all those who are weak and in need. They call us to greater compassion, kindness, and tenderness. They can teach us to become human.

I think Stanley Hauerwas' essay has got it right when he talks about L'Arche. The question is and always will be, how do we help our communities become and remain truly alive? How might we go about helping us all create a society where there is more love? How can we make a reality of our longed for vision of timeful friends?

REFERENCES

Beck, Martha. (2000) *Expecting Adam.* London: Judy Piatkus Ltd.
Ignatieff, Michael. (1985) *The Need of Strangers.* U.S.A.: Penquin Books.
Vanier, John. (1989) *Community and Growth.* London: Darton, Longman, and Todd.
(1999) *Becoming Human.* London: Darton, Longman, and Todd.
(2001) *Made for Happiness.* London: Darton, Longman, and Todd.

Response:
Making Yourself Useful

Michael Bérubé , PhD, MA, BA

SUMMARY. In this essay I reply to Stanley Hauerwas' reading of my book, *Life as We Know It*, by way of engaging Hauerwas' critique of Enlightenment humanism, and, more specifically, the Kantian categorical imperative. I argue that Hauerwas is mistaken to claim that "humanism cannot help but think that, all things considered, it would be better if [the mentally handicapped] did not exist," even as I agree in part with his trenchant critique of my own work and of the widely-accepted Kantian proposition that human beings should treat each other as ends in themselves, never as means to an end. Finally, I defend my antifoundationalist formulation of moral "obligation" with regard to persons with mental disabilities against Hauerwas's Christian critique thereof by noting that even Hauerwas, at a critical juncture of his argument, relies on a pragmatist, antifoundationalist understanding of what it means to "help" other humans–and what it means to make oneself useful. *[Article copies available for a fee from The Haworth Document Delivery Service: 1-800-HAWORTH. E-mail address: <docdelivery@haworthpress.com> Website: <http://www.Haworth Press.com> © 2004 by The Haworth Press, Inc. All rights reserved.]*

KEYWORDS. Disability, autonomy, dependency, humanism

Michael Bérubé is Paterno Family Professor in Literature, Pennsylvania University, and author of *The Employment of English: Theory, Jobs, and the Future of Literary Studies.* University Press: New York, 1998.

[Haworth co-indexing entry note]: "Response: Making Yourself Useful." Bérubé, Michael. Co-published simultaneously in *Journal of Religion, Disability & Health* (The Haworth Pastoral Press, an imprint of The Haworth Press, Inc.) Vol. 8, No. 3/4, 2004, pp. 31-36; and: *Critical Reflections on Stanley Hauerwas' Theology of Disability: Disabling Society, Enabling Theology* (ed: John Swinton) The Haworth Pastoral Press, an imprint of The Haworth Press, Inc., 2004, pp. 31-36. Single or multiple copies of this article are available for a fee from The Haworth Document Delivery Service [1-800-HAWORTH, 9:00 a.m. - 5:00 p.m. (EST). E-mail address: docdelivery@haworthpress.com].

Digital Object Identifier: 10.1300/J095v8n03_04

I must thank Stanley Hauerwas, first, for so invigorating a reading of my book; although it is a somewhat critical reading, it is also informed–or so it seems to me–by a spirit of caritas and a shared desire to remain open to the worlds, the signs, the desires, the lives of the mentally handicapped. Indeed, despite my secularist, anti-foundational foundations, I find myself in agreement with much of what Professor Hauerwas has to say–not only about my book, but about disability, autonomy, and modernity as well. I want to second Hauerwas' sense that "no group exposes the pretensions of the humanism that shapes the practices of modernity more thoroughly than the mentally handicapped"; I want to insist nonetheless that Hauerwas is wrong to argue that "the same humanism cannot help but think that, all things considered, it would be better if they did not exist"; and I want to confess that I, too, am haunted by the possibility that my writing about Jamie has simply "used" him to illustrate (and thereby try to advance) an intellectual and political agenda on matters ranging from language acquisition to the welfare state to theories of distributive justice.

First, however, I need to straighten out what appears to be a fundamental confusion about creatures. Hauerwas finds it "sad" that my sweetest dream for Jamie is that he will "someday be his own advocate, his own author, his own best representative," replying that

> [a]s Christians we know we have not been created to be 'our own authors,' to be autonomous. We are creatures. Dependency, not autonomy, is one of the ontological characteristics of our lives. That we are creatures, moreover, is but a reminder that we are created for and with one another. We are not just accidentally communal, but we are such by necessity. We were not created to be alone. We cannot help but desire and delight in the reality of the other, even the other born with a difference we call mentally handicapped.

This is an eloquent passage, as even we non-Christians will admit. And while Hauerwas is right to imagine that I would resist every invocation of our "created" beings and every speculation as to the purpose of our creation, he might be surprised to learn that I agree that dependency, not autonomy, is one of the ontological characteristics of our lives. I did not mean to suggest that Jamie could or should be utterly autonomous, his own self-designated deity; I meant (and mean) only that I hope Jamie grows up to be able to tell his own story, to learn to narrate his life to others. I mean "author" in a thoroughly secular sense, as a cognate of "advocate" and "representative," and I want Jamie to be his own author not only to assuage my intermittent guilt about "using" him for my own purposes, but also because there isn't anything I desire more ardently than for Jamie to be able to tell me about his day, about his trip to the park, about his new speech therapist, about how it feels to jump into the deep end of the pool, about why he wants to go to Hogwarts like Harry Potter, and about whether anyone at school or camp is mean to him.

As Professor Hauerwas knows, I argue at some length in *Life as We Know It* that the recognition of our fellow humans as fellow humans depends not on our innate, species-specific qualities or on our status as creatures of the divine will, but on quotidian, sublunary forms of political deliberation that make "recognition" of one's humanity a matter of embodied social policy. It is therefore all the more urgent, on my account, that persons with mental retardation be represented in the public square when they cannot represent themselves; and it is all the more urgent that persons with mental retardation who have long been presumed to be constitutively unable to represent themselves be granted the material means to represent themselves as best they can. If, as is likely, Jamie cannot be his own best representative, his own "author," in this secular sense, then he–like millions of persons with disabilities who cannot communicate any adequate and accurate sense of themselves to other people–will be all the more dependent on the intercession of others. The decisive thing is that those of us who identify ourselves, however temporarily, as "nondisabled" might come to understand Jamie's condition–autonomy as a regulative ideal for self-representation, dependency as the primary ontological fact of life–as exemplary rather than anomalous. If we humans can somehow come to such an understanding of our interdependent lives, then I will not haggle over whether Jamie should be understood as a *creature*, in Professor Hauerwas's sense, or as a mere secular *critter*, a kid who puts a slice of pizza in the microwave for three minutes and then comes upstairs to tell his father "I need help" when he sees smoke wafting through the kitchen. Jamie wants to be independent, to do it "all by *my*self," as he so often says; and it is incumbent on the rest of us to honor that desire even as we try to compensate for all the ways in which it will never quite be fulfilled.

I am, as the above paragraph attests, caught in a terrible paradox–affirming autonomy and dependency at once, and for different reasons. Surely Hauerwas is right to claim, à propos of my brief critique of Rawls, that my imagination reflects the same limits that formed the conceptions of justice I find so unsatisfactory. I am attempting to counter one post-Enlightenment narrative (the critique of utilitarianism launched by the Rawlsian account of distributive justice) by means of another (the critique of the Rawlsian "original position" launched by contemporary theorists of embodiment and disability): It is no wonder that I can so easily be hoisted on my own petard. Perhaps one of the lessons of my attempt to elaborate an antifoundationalist "ground" for intersubjective recognition is that no one post-Enlightenment narrative of humanity will suffice. It could also be the case that my attempt simply wasn't good enough: After all, despite my best efforts, I wound up crafting an argument that, in its conclusion, subtly reinstates a communication-based performance criterion for being human–as parents of and advocates for people with autism and severe and profound retardation have kindly pointed out to me.

Still, I think there is no reason for Hauerwas to claim that the post-Enlightenment, antifoundationalist humanism I have tried to imagine is a humanism that, in its private moments, breaks down, puts its head in its hands, and confesses that "it would be better" if persons with mental retardation did not exist. I simply do not see how the claim follows from anything I have written or professed; I am not even sure what this "it" is that would possibly be "better" in a world divested of the frailties of flesh. Does Professor Hauerwas imagine that disabilities are a burden to humanism, or merely that some able-bodied humanists of allegedly sound mind sometimes imagine that people with disabilities would be better off without their disabilities? It is possible to argue that one brutally reductive strain of Enlightenment thought led the West to the massive folly of eugenics, but the humanism I know and love is a humanism that does not believe in the perfectibility of the species and does not presume to say what forms of embodiment would be "better" for all concerned.

By contrast, Hauerwas mounts a useful (for lack of a still more pointed word) critique of Enlightenment humanism when he uses the phenomenon of mental retardation to argue against Kant's second formulation of the categorical imperative: Even though I will, once again, refrain from saying that we were "put" here or that we were "put" here in order "to be of use to one another," I will confess that Hauerwas' critique of Kant, and of Kant's profound influence on moral theory (evidenced by the fact that "we cannot imagine anyone seriously challenging it as a statement of what we should at least always try to do"), brought me to realize that I had not fully thought through my reliance on the idea that humans should regard each other as ends rather than means. Hauerwas writes: "The notion that any use we make of one another can only be justified if it is done voluntarily can now be seen as one of the peculiar sentimentalities of modernity that results in self-supervision all the more tyrannical since what we do is allegedly what we want to do." Reading those lines with a sharp intake of breath, I remembered that toward the end of *Life as We Know It*, I had written (in a passage that Professor Hauerwas is too generous to cite) that "I hope none of us was put here for the benefit of others." I meant, at the time, to register my revulsion at the idea that people with Down syndrome (for instance) are "put here" to humanize the rest of us, but I realize now that my aversion to the human uses of human beings was perhaps too fastidious. Professor Hauerwas is right: In the course of our lives we cannot not make use of others, and how awful would it be, in ethical theory or in family gatherings, if we did not set out making ourselves *useful* to others?

The problem lies, of course, in determining what constitutes a "good" use of another human being. It is one thing to make oneself useful, and quite another to make of other humans mere instruments of one's will. How then, can the non-Christian make sense of Hauerwas's pivotal anti-Kantian claim?

> As Christians we should not feel embarrassed to discover that the mentally handicapped among us help us better understand the narrative that constitutes the very purpose of our existence. That such is the case does not "justify" their existence, but then their existence no more than our existence from a Christian perspective requires justification. *We are free to help them just to the extent we no longer feel the necessity to justify their existence*. The form such "help" takes can only be discovered relative to the tasks of the community necessary to sustain the practices for the discovery and care of the goods held in common (my emphasis).

I have emphasized the third sentence above because I think it is the pivot within the pivot, the bridge between the words Hauerwas writes as part of a fellowship of Christians (in the first two sentences) and the words he writes to define "help" (it is crucial, is it not, that at the crux of the problem of "help" Hauerwas must write "help" in scare quotes) in what are ultimately pragmatist, antifoundationalist terms. As Christians, Professor Hauerwas writes, we learn that the mentally handicapped help us, and that we may help them to the degree that we are no longer required to justify their existence (this latter clause, by the way, is a brilliant and wonderful formulation); but when it comes to asking whether our own attempts to "help" them are indeed helpful, then we cannot claim sanction from a narrative of divine intention, and must fall back instead to the task of defining "help" relative to the tasks of a community necessary to sustain the practices for the discovery and care of the goods held in common. This is a modest, pragmatist, and indeterminate conclusion–and, I believe, an appropriate one.

As non-Christians, if I may presume to speak for or to some of them in closing, we therefore find a place in Hauerwas's model, a place where we, too, can be of use–as defined relative to the tasks of a community–precisely to the extent that we do not feel compelled to justify the existence of the mentally handicapped. In *Life as We Know It* I tried to argue that we have obligations to others and that these obligations have no other basis than our ability to imagine them; but I suppose I was still too anxious, or too conflicted, or insufficiently antifoundationalist, to forego the attempt to justify the ways of Jamie Bérubé to man. This time I will try to eschew justification altogether, and in doing so I will echo Professor Hauerwas's and Jean Vanier's words on friend-ship by quoting something Jamie said to me last month as he fell asleep on my arm while we were riding a train to New York. "Daddy," he said, groggily and with reference to nothing at all, "always be my friend." As I assured him, with all my heart, that I would always be his friend, I couldn't help wondering, *now, where in the world did that come from*? Thanks to Hauerwas and Vanier, I now know I need not bother asking. The question, like the fact of our obligations to each other, does not "come from" anywhere. It is simply here, now that Jamie is here, and the only thing that matters is that Christians and non-Christians alike respond to it with all the caritas they can invent or imagine.

Chapter 2

Community and Diversity: The Tyranny of Normality

Stanley Hauerwas, PhD

[From *Suffering Presence: Theological Reflections on Medicine, the Mentally Handicapped, and the Church*. 1986, pp. 211-217. Originally a talk delivered at the 1977 annual dinner of the Council for the Retarded of St. Joseph County, Indiana.] Reprinted with permission.

SUMMARY. Hauerwas explores dimensions of the question: 'what is normal.' Exploring the ideas of normality and difference he offers a critique of the 'principle of normality.' What is normality? Normality as it is often formulated can be dangerous for people with developmental disabilities. 'The most stringent power we have over another is not physical coercion but the ability to have another accept our definition of them.' Hauerwas argues that what is required is not a common norm but a form of community which respects diversity and seeks to enable each member to accept the 'gift of differentness,' and to accept that difference without regret.

[Haworth co-indexing entry note]: "Community and Diversity: The Tyranny of Normality." Hauerwas, Stanley. Co-published simultaneously in *Journal of Religion, Disability & Health* (The Haworth Pastoral Press, an imprint of The Haworth Press, Inc.) Vol. 8, No. 3/4, 2004, pp. 37-43; and: *Critical Reflections on Stanley Hauerwas' Theology of Disability: Disabling Society, Enabling Theology* (ed: John Swinton) The Haworth Pastoral Press, an imprint of The Haworth Press, Inc., 2004, pp. 37-43. Single or multiple copies of this article are available for a fee from The Haworth Document Delivery Service [1-800-HAWORTH, 9:00 a.m. - 5:00 p.m. (EST). E-mail address: docdelivery@haworthpress.com].

http://www.haworthpress.com/web/JRDH
Digital Object Identifier: 10.1300/J095v8n03_05

KEYWORDS. Difference, normality, community, acceptance, power, definition

It is a great honor for me to be given the opportunity to speak at such an occasion. For I have no claim or right to be heard by you. Those of you who have retarded children and/or work with retarded children already know far more than anything I could say. Moreover, you have felt the sadness, suffering, and joy of being, having, and working with retarded citizens that I have not. It is an honor that you have asked me to speak to you, since I feel that day in and day out you speak much more eloquently to me.

Therefore, I must speak to you as an "outsider" who has had the privilege of being with those on the inside. Usually there is not much advantage to being an "outsider," but at least it gives me the opportunity to see what you are doing through fresh eyes. For I have noticed that those who have retarded children and work with the retarded are often so busy doing, they have little time to reflect on why, how, or what they are doing. This is, of course, not an unusual thing to have happen. It has been remarked that if fish ever developed intelligence and began to codify and describe their environment, one of the last things they would notice would be the water. Therefore, as an outsider, I want to try to say a few things tonight that may help you notice what kind of water you folks are swimming in, in terms of that which binds us together–namely, our commitment to the support of those born not like us that we describe with the unhappy word "retarded."

Now I am bold enough to take this tack because I think that one of our difficulties is that you do not know how to describe why it is that we share this commitment. In other words, I think that our culture too often offers us no account, or worse–a misleading account, of this commitment. Each of you has developed your special, or perhaps better, your personal account of why this commitment is so significant. Such accounts often are as profoundly simple as what it means to be a parent or they may involve convictions about one's own vocation. But as important as our personal accounts are, we need more if the existence and care of the retarded are to be seen as important for the outsider. We need an account that helps give, not only those involved with the retarded, but also those who only support that involvement indirectly, a sense that this is a good and essential task for everyone in our community.

Moreover, when we lack such accounts or stories about what we are doing, we often are captured by destructive accounts. On the personal level, for example, we can tell ourselves false stories about being sacrificial parents–to the detriment of our children. We know this is dangerous because we learn how hard it is to make a sacrifice without making those we sacrificed for pay for our effort. Or we can be captured by destructive accounts about the retarded–namely, they are more innocent or sweet than other children or people. That is a terrible story to have to live out, because who wants to go through life being innocent and sweet?

At a social level we also can run into some misleading claims about what we are doing. For example, many of us fighting for better treatment for the retarded use the language of securing the rights of the retarded. To be sure, the language of rights has a moral and social significance, but we must use it carefully, for too often in our political system it is the battle cry of one group against another. When used in this manner it transforms what should be this society's moral commitment into an issue comparable to a conflict between businesses and labor. If we are to use the language of rights, we must do so only as a means to protect the retarded from those who would treat them, for either cruel or sentimental reasons, with less than respect.

I think it is important, therefore, that we remember that the language of rights is dependent on a more profound sense of community that forms our commitment to the retarded. Speaking as the "outsider," I want to suggest that the retarded help us understand some crucial things about what it means to be a community that enhances us all. Put differently, many talks about the retarded are about what we should be doing for them, but I am suggesting that they do something for us that we have hardly noticed. Namely, they force us to recognize that we are involved in a community life that is richer than our official explanations and theories give us the skill to say.

For example, we usually associate movements towards justice in our society with the language of equality. We assume to be treated equally is to be treated justly, but on reflection we may discover that is not the case. Often the language of equality only works by reducing us to a common denominator that can be repressive or disrespectful. This can perhaps be seen most clearly in terms of the black struggle for civil rights. That struggle began with a justified call to be treated equally–to have the opportunity to enjoy the same rights of all Americans that blacks were denied on the basis of their color. But, black Americans soon discovered that it was not enough to be treated equally if that treatment meant they must forget what it means to be black. Being black is just who they are. To be "black" is to be part of a history that should be cherished and enhanced. Noone wants to pay the price of being treated equally if that means they must reject who they are–that is, if they must reject their roots. We find the same kind of movement today among those born Hungarian, Spanish, or (the ultimate good) Texan. In other words, none of us want to be treated equally if that means we lose our distinctiveness.

Now it seems to me that our commitment to having the retarded in our society embodies a richer sense of community than the language of equality provides. For the retarded, in a profounder way than being black, Hungarian, Pole, or even Texan, call us toward a community of diversity and difference. Such a community is a community of equality, but not in the way that equality makes us forget our differences. Rather in a community of equality our differences help each of us to flourish exactly as different people.

There should be no mistake about it, a community of diversity that enhances differences is indeed a hard enterprise to sustain. We are creatures that fear difference. The fact that the other is not as we are means that there may be something wrong with us. The only solution is to make them as much like us as possible or to make them live apart. Most of us learn to deal with this demand to be like everyone else—we have the power. It should be said, however, that we are not nearly as successful as we think, as too often we voluntarily accept the other's definition of them. The most stringent power we have over another is not physical coercion but the ability to have the other accept our definition of them. But the retarded are often in the unfortunate position of not having the power to resist those who would make them like us.

This consideration, I think, must make us a little cautious about being too enthusiastic about the "principle of normalization" that is currently so popular among those who work with the retarded. It is of course true that the retarded deserve to do what they are able–to dress themselves, to spend their own money, to decide to spend their money foolishly or wisely, to date, to fall in love, and so on. But the demand to be normal can be tyrannical unless we understand that the normal condition of our being together is that we are all different. If we are to be a good community we must be one that has convictions substantive enough not to fear our differences and, indeed to see that we would not be whole without the other being different than us.

Besides the gift of difference and its importance for community, it seems to me that the retarded also help us to see how to be different without regret. It is one of the conditions of modern consciousness that we feel that we have suffered injustice or that we are ruled by powers not of our own making. Put graphically, we all tend to think of ourselves, at least in some moods, as victims.

Now I suspect that we have all in one way or another suffered injustice, but there is a problem with thinking of ourself as a victim. Because once we take on that role it may make us misdescribe what our problem is and we look for help in the wrong place. It makes us acquiesce too readily to our condition, assuming that there is nothing we can do until something is done out there.

On anyone's scale of those who have suffered some of the worst injustices across human societies, surely the retarded would be close to the top. But by what must almost be considered special grace, they do not think of themselves as victims. And I do not think that this is simply because they fail to understand what has happened to them. Rather it seems to me that they understand that we all get "stuck with" certain limits and certain societies. I am "stuck with" being a Texan and being bald, but the question is what I am going to do with being so "stuck." To be sure, some social conditions make some things we are "stuck with" unjust, and we ought not to tolerate that. But finally we must all learn, as it seems to me that the retarded often do better than any of us, that ultimately we are all "stuck with" ourselves, and that is not a bad thing.

For the limits we are "stuck with" are as much a source of our difference as are our talents. We are valuable to one another, not in spite of our talents, but because of them. Even though the retarded represent a limit in our communities, they also represent a limit we cannot be without. For without them and the attitude they bring to their limits, we would all be the poorer.

For example, let me suggest what I have observed the retarded have done for their parents. First, they have required their parents to join together and come in contact with others who are as different from them as their own children. In the process they discover they have interests beyond simply sharing similar children. They share similar pains and sufferings, joy, and triumphs that join them in community more profound than a mere association. That is the reason they can risk disagreement, because they know they are bound together in profound and lasting ways.

Secondly, parents of retarded children discover what the world is like through their children. Their children provide them with the means to break through the myths and illusions that our social order wants us to accept–namely, that life is about being members of the Pepsi® generation. Or society encourages us to think that one can be a good people without suffering, that we can pursue our own interests with little thought of what it does to others. But parents of children born retarded know better. No people in society can be good without paying a price. The crucial thing is how we help and support one another as we are each called upon to pay that price.

Or on a more mundane, but no less important level, I have noticed the parents of retarded children know a lot more about politics than most of us. You know who your state congress person is and you know how to get in touch with her or him. You know the institutions that sustain and run us and you learn how to make them work for the good. Without your children you would be just as uninformed as the average American about the social system that forms our lives.

Finally, one of the things your children have done for you is to help you be free from the tyranny of the professional. Now this involves arduous training and struggle that is never over, but generally you do better at it than most of us. For example, almost no one in our society has the guts to ask doctors for a second opinion, but you do. You have learned to do that because you have learned that professionals can be wrong and you are not going to let your child suffer because of the ego of a professional.

In fact, what parents of retarded children learn to do is trust their own good judgment, and that is a hard thing to do in a society which assumes that there is an expert for everything. We all need help from one another, but not because some are "experts" and others are not, but because good communities learn to use the experience that comes from different functions. But we must remember that when it comes to our children we are all experts and we should not let a professional determine what our child is, means, or can do.

Now I have been speaking as an outsider, but in closing I think it best to let an insider speak. In a book called *Journey*, Suzanne and Robert Massie describe their struggle to keep alive and raise their hemophilic son (source not referenced in original text). Mrs. Massie, pregnant with her third child, discovers the development and increasing accuracy of prenatal diagnosis. And of course the question arises whether she would have welcomed such counseling before the birth of her hemophilic son. She says,

> Perhaps, even very soon, premarital genetic counseling will be routine. No doubt this will be useful and helpful. But I couldn't help thinking as I heard those discussions among doctors, how glad I was that I had not been counseled BEFORE. For one thing, it is such an uneven relationship–the doctor, wearing a white coat and radiating scientific superiority, advising an untechnical, uninformed, frightened lay person. There is little training for such counseling in medical schools today–doctors are left to their own prejudices. Much of what passes under the guise of medical counselling really consists only of saying no; of advising the safe way, the way of least resistance. Not long ago, I attended a medical symposium and heard a famous geneticist talk learnedly about the need for "objective" counseling in cases of genetic disease. Fine. Then he concluded his remarks with this highly subjective sentence: "I cannot imagine a family who would not WISH TO AVOID the emotional and financial stress imposed upon them when a hemophiliac is born."

> I wonder. Suppose someone had talked to me this way? Suppose I had been told before I was married that I was a carrier for hemophilia and therefore should not have any children? Suppose I had been advised to adopt children? Personally, I am profoundly grateful that I was not told,

that I did not have to make the decision of whether to have or not to have Bobby. Looking back at myself, a newly married young woman, unfamiliar with the feelings of a mother, I think, had I been asked, I would have said no. No one wants to suffer. Everyone is afraid of challenge and sacrifice. This is normal and known. If someone had asked me, "Do you want to walk through fire?" the answer would have been no, of course not. I am afraid of being burned. Yet once in the fire, I fought to get through it and it is at least possible to think that the experience left me stronger. It is not the struggle but the unknown that we fear most. If genetic counseling is to be meaningful, then not only must those counseled be informed of the purely scientific facts, they must also be encouraged to believe in themselves, in their own capacities to live and grow. They must be counseled not only to FEAR, but to be brave enough to live with the question.

Without questions, would we ever search for answers? A child with a genetic illness is a perpetual question, pushing us to seek answers to this dilemma of nature and God. It was with all these vivid impressions that I waited for my third child. I can add nothing to this, for if an "outsider" is wise he should know when to shut up and let the "insiders" speak. But what I hope I have at least suggested is that the struggle, the pain, the suffering, and the joy of the "insiders" is not insignificant for those of us on the outside. For without you and your children, our communities would be less rich in the diversity of folk that we need in order to be good communities.

Response:
Whose Table for "The Retarded"?

John O'Brien

SUMMARY. They key role of those treated as outsiders in building community is identified. The importance of appreciating people with intellectual disabilities as possessing affirmative gifts and the necessity of understanding "outsiders" through sharing life is asserted. The centrality of dependency in understanding community building and the positive historical role of the principle of normalization in highlighting the negative effects of segregation and control are discussed. *[Article copies available for a fee from The Haworth Document Delivery Service: 1-800-HAWORTH. E-mail address: <docdelivery@haworthpress.com> Website: <http://www.HaworthPress.com> © 2004 by The Haworth Press, Inc. All rights reserved.]*

KEYWORDS. Community building, mental retardation, normalization, l'Arche, citizen advocacy

John O'Brien has worked extensively with people with disabilities. For the past 25 years, he and Connie Lyle O'Brien have cooperated with a network of people to build local capacity to include people with substantial disabilities in all aspects of community life.

[Haworth co-indexing entry note]: "Response: Whose Table for 'The Retarded'?" O'Brien, John. Co-published simultaneously in *Journal of Religion, Disability & Health* (The Haworth Pastoral Press, an imprint of The Haworth Press, Inc.) Vol. 8, No. 3/4, 2004, pp. 45-51; and: *Critical Reflections on Stanley Hauerwas' Theology of Disability: Disabling Society, Enabling Theology* (ed: John Swinton) The Haworth Pastoral Press, an imprint of The Haworth Press, Inc., 2004, pp. 45-51. Single or multiple copies of this article are available for a fee from The Haworth Document Delivery Service [1-800-HAWORTH, 9:00 a.m. - 5:00 p.m. (EST). E-mail address: docdelivery@haworthpress.com].

http://www.haworthpress.com/web/JRDH
© 2004 by The Haworth Press, Inc. All rights reserved.
Digital Object Identifier: 10.1300/J095v8n03_06

In the past 30 years I have often eaten my portion of the casserole before rising to address the annual meeting of an association that supports people with intellectual disabilities. Noticing in a footnote that Stanley Hauerwas delivered this paper as a talk in a similar setting opened my way into his wise and puzzling contribution. As I imagined Hauerwas's words in the familiar setting of a celebratory meal I wondered, "That night, who shared the table with these people he calls 'the retarded' and who, to Hauerwas's way of thinking, was missing?"

The paper's wisdom needs no interpretation. We are called to the difficult work of creating good communities. Good communities include diversity and difference based on a conviction that we cannot be whole without others being different from us; in such communities people can be different without regret. In building good communities we must act from conviction deep enough to overcome our fear of difference and safeguard our temptation to either separate those who carry frightening differences away from us or attempt to discipline them into simulacra of a tame and bland normality. The prevalence of thin, impoverished, ahistorical, and misleading accounts of difference in relationship to society, community, and family makes forming the necessary conviction difficult. The language of rights and the language of equality are not sufficient to carry us as far as we need to go toward communities that enhance us all. People with mental retardation have an important, if easily ignored, role in deepening the conviction that sustains community sufficiently to keep the language of rights and the language of equality in their proper context: They call us out of too thin official explanations and theories and quietly confront us with differing gifts.

This summary is not, of course, Hauerwas's message. The message is the story he told about "the retarded" to the assembled parents and workers who "have felt the sadness, suffering, and joy of being, having, and working with retarded citizens." It is in following the shape and turnings of that story that I grow puzzled. In thinking about my puzzlement I identify three differences with this paper: (1) its account of the potential gifts of people with intellectual disabilities is too thin; (2) consequently its call to community is too weak; and (3) it has too limited an understanding of the way modern projects, like implementing the principle of normalization, can open spaces for the Holy Spirit's work.

The quotation marks surrounding "the retarded" are not a postmodern gesture but the fruit of counsel offered by my friend, Peter Park, who has lived his whole life with the consequences of being understood and treated in terms of the label, including spending 18 years in an institution for "the retarded" after his parents followed professional advice to place him there. Peter abhors the word as an enemy of the kinds of relationships that he and I believe are fundamental signs that the Spirit is at work slowly building a decent and diverse community. "Retarded," Peter advised, "was the excuse for putting us in institutions, for sterilizing us, for keeping us without any real work to do, for putting us in time-out cells and restraints because we didn't do what staff told us quick enough to suit them. It's even the excuse people like Doctor Singer use for saying it would be good to kill us as babies (Singer & Kuhse, 1985). If you have to write the word because somebody else did, at least put marks around it and remind them of the harm it has done us."

WHO ARE "THE RETARDED" TO HAUERWAS?

Hauerwas begins his talk by defining himself as "an outsider," lacking the right to be heard by those who have or work with "those born not like us that we describe with the unhappy word 'retarded.' " Because this claim to outsider status survived the collection of the talk into a book, it deserves consideration as more than a rhetorical move: does it name a distance between himself and "the retarded"? Based only on this text, I think it does, and I think this distance thins his account of the gifts people with intellectual disabilities can bring to building community.

Four out of five things "the retarded" do for the rest of us arise from what Hauerwas says having them has done for their parents: "The retarded" have bound their parents into association with others who are different from themselves beyond the fact of sharing what he calls similar children; they have taught their parents that life without suffering is illusory but that suffering can be the basis for help and support (here I am uncertain but I think he is talking about the suffering of the parents and the help and support they offer one another rather than about the suffering of "the retarded" and the help and support that they offer); their presence has caused their parents to become more politically informed and active than the average citizen; and they have freed their parents from deference to experts. What interests me about this list is not its overgeneralization of the qualities parents display–e.g., many hundreds of parents would tell a story of deferring to experts in institutionalizing their children–but the passivity of "the retarded" in the process. As best I can understand him, Hauerwas thinks that simply by being "the retarded" they engender in their parents the sadness, suffering, and joy that parents, in association, turn into a kind of community that can resist at least some of the temptations of the Enlightenment. This argument seems to me to have many steps missing.

The fifth contribution of "the retarded"is to model acceptance of personal and social limitations, even to the point of suffering injustice without resentment. This gift arises from "a special grace" that frees "the retarded" from thinking of themselves as victims, though they suffer some of the worst of society's injustices. This grace allows them to understand that we all get "stuck with" certain limitations. I have been taught much by the fact that many people with significant cognitive differences do communicate a deep sense of wholeness to those with eyes to see and ears to hear. But the notion that rejection and exclusion do not wound and stunt "the retarded" is simply a nonsense that would put "the retarded" somehow above or outside the need for the same church that the rest of us sinners are called to count on.

Jean Vanier (2001; 1998), another Aristotelian, provides a more provocative account of the gifts of people with intellectual disabilities. He left his philosophy teaching job in 1964 to live in a faith-founded community based on sharing everyday life and seeking friendship among people with and without intellectual disabilities. He did so because, with the support of his spiritual accompanier, Father Thomas, he heard the call to live community from Raphael and Philippe, two institutionalized men. In their life together, these four men called others and their household has seeded many small communities where disabled and non-disabled people struggle to practice the virtues in common.

Vanier expresses a clearer sense of the daily consequences of the wounds that many people with disabilities suffer because others do not relate to them as even potential friends. Therefore he communicates a deeper sense of people's unique and ordinary gifts, given the chance to struggle with the continual imperfections of a journeying community founded on the possibility of friendship. His is not a romantic account. "Community is the place where are revealed all the darkness and anger, jealousies, and rivalry hidden in our hearts" (Vanier, 1992, p. 29), he says, drawing no distinction between disabled and non-disabled community members. But it is exactly in sharing weakness and need, in telling and hearing each other's stories, in forgiving and asking forgiveness over and again, in holding one another to account for living up to common agreements that Vanier (1999, p. 89) can say "people with intellectual disabilities brought me more into my body . . . [and] led me from a serious world into a world of celebration, presence, and laughter: the world of the heart."

WHOSE COMMUNITY?

It is hard to tell from this text who Hauerwas wants to call to consciousness as a community, largely because the pronouns keep sliding around. Most often he calls forth a "you" that binds parents or parents and staff together. Sometimes the parent-staff "you" becomes an "us" in which the speaker slips from his outsider status. He does not seem to directly address "the retarded" as listening, acting members of "us" (indeed I wonder how many people with disabilities shared the meal at which he spoke). Beyond counseling restraint in appeals to rights, and suggesting that outsiders should know how supporting "the retarded" matters to everyone, Hauerwas does not ask his listeners to imagine how to make their "you" bigger, to include more current outsiders in the direct and personal involvement in relationship with the people with intellectual disabilities who offer important benefits to their parents and staff. By the time Hauerwas talked, seven years experience with citizen advocacy–focused efforts to build relationships between intellectually disabled people and ordinary citizens–had demonstrated the practical possibility, and the difficulty of constructing a more capacious "you" (O'Brien & Lyle O'Brien, 1996).

Hauerwas does not invite his listeners to recognize and struggle to transform those habits and practices of their daily life that allow him to place himself in the outsider role. He does not ask his listeners to consider how to move beyond the separating out of "the retarded" as a group that draw the limits of human community, maybe in part because he has a notion that "the retarded" are somehow a distinct human group, like Hungarians or Texans, he says. This analogy defines overcoming fear of difference as the problem and might lead to the thought that some form of tolerance will suffice to build community. This could be true for Texans in general, but I think it oversimplifies the issue for Texans with intellectual disabilities. And I think the oversimplification matters because it underestimates the role of God's grace in sustaining the hard work of building community.

In my experience, personal contact often dissolves the perception of difference that separates people on the basis of intellectual disability; unusual movements, unique ways of communicating, strange appearances, and obvious limits in learning often fade when people meet each other in almost any ordinary setting. What does not dissolve is the reality of dependence: This person needs specific and unusual assistance or accommodation from most others every single day. The asymmetry generated by dependence continually tempts those who offer assistance and those who receive it to freeze themselves into postures of power and dependency that obscure gifts and distract from taking the next steps in a shared journey. I think that the most frightening reality that people with intellectual disabilities raise is the difficulty of living gracefully with the continuing demands and temptations of practical dependency. The illusion they confront, an illusion that is often tangible enough to keep them segregated with "their own kind," is the idol of individual self-sufficiency.

Absent the chance of being touched in the heart by someone who has seemed frighteningly different and remains dependent, it is doubtful that the community Hauerwas points toward will have much chance of becoming real. If Hauerwas wants his listeners to imagine needing a few more place settings each year to feed the slowly growing numbers of former outsiders who come to the table because they count people with disabilities as friends, he is shy to say so here. If he knows that the Holy Spirit must have room to work in order to sustain a community that makes friendship possible despite difference and dependence, he is shy to say so here.

Reconsidering Normalization

Hauerwas urges caution about enthusiasm for the principle of normalization. My friends and I experienced normalization in the 1970s as a resource for groping our way along our journey toward decent relationships with people we held power over, a journey that did not end as our ability to express its guiding principles left the easily misunderstood word, normalization, to a cherished place in our history. Hauerwas apparently takes normalization to be a mix of two things. One of these things he approves of, allowing "the retarded" do what they are able in the way of dressing, dating, spending money and other typical activities. The other he and I see as deeply dangerous: attempting to make "the retarded" normal (whatever Enlightenment nightmare that may be) and thus stripping them of differences important to their identity and history. This could have been what he heard and saw of normalization in South Bend, but he settled for a shallow take on the hard practical and conceptual work that was going on in many places in North America in the 1970s.

A history of the idea of normalization up to the date of Hauerwas's talk is found in Wolfensberger (1999, pp. 51-116) in a book whose multiple contributors bring some of the story into the mid-1990s. Peter Park (1999, pp. 475-476), my friend and advisor quoted above, reflects in this volume on the way the principle of normalization has influenced his 61 years of life with a label. He develops his understanding of the relationship between honest efforts to follow the principle of normalization and having what he calls "more diverse communities where people with different abilities can learn from each other."

None of this detracts from the prudence of Hauerwas' suspicions. The principle of normalization expresses the Enlightenment project in just the same way that the association that invited him to give this talk does. Without a deeper sense of community language of rights and the language of equality. But such is the power of the Spirit that honest attempts to live and work even in its modern terms have sometimes set the conditions for friendships to emerge that take their participants another few steps toward that community that enhances us all.

REFERENCES

Kuhse, H., & Singer, P. (1985). *Should the Baby Live? The Problem of Handicapped Infants.* Oxford: Oxford University Press.

O'Brien, J., & Lyle O'Brien, C. (1996). *Members of each other: Building community in company with people with developmental disabilities.* Toronto, ON: Inclusion Press.

Park, P., & French, B. (1999). The impact of normalization on my life. In R. Flynn & R. LeMay, eds. *A quarter-century of normalization and social role valorization: Evolution and impact.* Ottawa, ON: University of Ottawa Press.

Vanier, J. (2001). *Made for happiness: Discovering the meaning of life with Aristotle.* Toronto, ON: House of Anansi Press.

Vanier, J. (1998). *Becoming human: The CBC Massey Lectures.* Toronto, ON: House of Anansi Press.

Vanier, J. (1992). *From brokenness to community. The Wit Lectures at Harvard Divinity School.* New York: Paulist Press.

Wolfensberger, W. (1999). A contribution to the history of normalization, with primary emphasis on the establishment of normalization in North America between 1967-1975. In R. Flynn & R. LeMay, Eds. *A quarter-century of normalization and social role valorization: Evolution and impact.* Ottawa, ON: University of Ottawa Press.

Chapter 3

The Church and the Mentally Handicapped: A Continuing Challenge to the Imagination

Stanley Hauerwas, PhD

SUMMARY. In this essay Hauerwas explores the experience of children with developmental disabilities and their parents. Arguing against the problemitization of disability Hauerwas asks the piercing question: What are children *for*? He presents a case for suggesting that the 'problems' that children with developmental disabilities encounter are not inherent within their condition, but rather are created by the type of society that they inhabit and the assumptions about the purpose of children within such a society. Whilst society tends to treat children as commodities which can be picked and chosen according to personal desire, Hauerwas presents

[Haworth co-indexing entry note]: "The Church and the Mentally Handicapped: A Continuing Challenge to the Imagination." Hauerwas, Stanley. Co-published simultaneously in *Journal of Religion, Disability & Health* (The Haworth Pastoral Press, an imprint of The Haworth Press, Inc.) Vol. 8, No. 3/4, 2004, pp. 53-62; and: *Critical Reflections on Stanley Hauerwas' Theology of Disability: Disabling Society, Enabling Theology* (ed: John Swinton) The Haworth Pastoral Press, an imprint of The Haworth Press, Inc., 2004, pp. 53-62. Single or multiple copies of this article are available for a fee from The Haworth Document Delivery Service [1-800-HAWORTH, 9:00 a.m. - 5:00 p.m. (EST). E-mail address: docdelivery@haworthpress.com].

a case for a theological understanding of parenting which locates responsibility for the individual child firmly within the Christian community. Children are signs of hope in the midst of a dark world. To have a child is a profound act of faith. Children, whether disabled or otherwise, are *gifts* given to the community. The church is constituted by those people who can take the time in a world crying with injustice to accept these Graceful gifts, some of whom may turn out to be developmentally disabled.

KEYWORDS. Disabled children, the church, community, imagination

THE "PROBLEM" OF "THE PROBLEM"
OF THE MENTALLY HANDICAPPED

The challenge of being as well as caring for those called "mentally handicapped" is to prevent those who wish they never existed or would "just go away" from defining them as "the problem" of the mentally handicapped. It is almost impossible to resist descriptions that make being mentally handicapped "a problem," since those descriptions are set by the power of the "normal." For example, parents who have a mentally handicapped child often were and sometimes still are told that such a child will be happier "institutionalized." Such roadblocks continue when parents try to get adequate medical care and often find that doctors assume it would be better for everyone if this child would die. The adversity continues as parents face the hundreds of silent slights contained in the stares of people in grocery stores and service stations, stares that communicate–"thank God that is not me."

Such roadblocks and slights are destined to get worse as our society seeks and finds ways to eliminate the mentally handicapped. What will happen, for example, if this society starts requiring amniocentesis? The human genome project is a potential threat to the mentally handicapped as it will encourage the presumption that people should regulate their sexual and marital behavior to avoid having handicapped children. What will our society say to those who decide to challenge the presuppositions that we ought to avoid having mentally handicapped children? It is possible to envision that society may well put legal and financial penalties on people who decide to have children who are less than "normal."

Of course, implicit in these projects is the false assumption that most of the mentally handicapped are primarily born rather than made. Thus, even if this society decides to eliminate the birth of mentally handicapped children, they will continue to be confronted by those who are environmentally handicapped, that is, those whose condition is the result of pollution, nutritional deficits, and poverty rather than genetics. The care of those children whose handicaps result from such environmental causes may be even worse, since on the whole this society already has decided that such "unfortunate accidents" should not exist.

There are, moreover, roadblocks interfering with adequate training of the mentally handicapped. Schools are not set up to handle mentally handicapped people because such individuals do not learn as we learn. Mentally handicapped folks are segregated, not because they cannot learn, but because they are segregated for being not like us. Furthermore, we fear those who are not like us. It is said that they will slow other children down, and well they might, but it is never thought that they might morally speed up other children.

Faced with such obstacles and challenges, those who have and care for the mentally handicapped often feel their most immediate task is to try to overcome the immediate threats to the mentally handicapped. They become advocates of normalization and fight for the "least restrictive alternatives" for the mentally handicapped. These strategies, to be sure, have much to recommend them, but too easily they can become part of the agenda of those who basically want to deny the existence of the mentally handicapped. Ask yourself, for example, would you want to be pressured to be normal? Who is to say what that entails? Since I am a Texan I would not have the slightest idea what it means to be normal. While I do not disagree with most of the recommendations put forward in the name of normalization, I do worry that that concept does not in itself specify what we need to say on behalf of the mentally handicapped; or perhaps better put, it does not focus on what we need to make possible for the mentally handicapped to say on their own behalf.

Particularly disturbing are the ways in which our confrontation of the challenges facing the mentally handicapped tend to put the burden of care entirely on the family. Our society seems to say, "Your luck was bad, and now you are stuck with this kid. We will help you so long as you do not ask for too much." Therefore, the family becomes the only agent representing the mentally handicapped, since absolutely no one else is there to represent them.

Many who care for the mentally handicapped then get caught up in contradictions that seem unavoidable. For example, in the interest of supporting families in their care of the mentally handicapped, often against unfeeling bureaucracies, we maintain that families have all rights regarding the mentally handicapped. The family can serve the interest of the child on the assumption that parents best know the child's needs.

However, we then feel at a loss when we encounter families who do not want to care for the child. Those who refuse to provide basic medical care for a Downs Syndrome baby who needs further surgery is only one dramatic example. As a result, we have institutions filled with mentally handicapped people who are there because they have been abandoned by the only people this society thinks can care for them—their parents.

The Mentally Handicapped and the Christian Imagination

These examples challenge our imaginations concerning how we are to act with the mentally handicapped. What has gone wrong is not that we lack goodwill, but that we simply do not know how to care because we need the challenge of real people who will teach us how to care. Such people really are the imagination of a community, for we must remember that imagination is not something we have in our minds. Rather, the imagination is a pattern of possibilities fostered within a community by the stories and correlative commitments that make it what it is. Necessities force us out of our paths of least resistance, and, as a result, they make us more likely to form communities that know how to care for one another.

Our imaginations, when driven by little more than the logic of our desires, easily can lead us astray. As Christians, this fact should not surprise us, since we have learned that those aspects of our lives that offer the greatest resources for good also offer equivalent resources for evil. This is why human imagination, like any other human capacity, must be ordered by something more determinative.

For Christians, that something is both the story of who God has called us to be and our concrete attempts to faithfully embody that calling. For a community with such a self-understanding, imagination is not a power that somehow exists "in the mind"; instead, it is a pointer to a community's constant willingness to expose itself to the innovations required by its convictions about who God is. Similarly, the world is seen differently when construed by such an imaginative community, for the world is not simply there, always ready to be known, but rather is known well only when known through the practices and habits of a community constituted by a truthful story.

The Christian imagination forces us to acknowledge that the world is different from what it seems. That difference requires Christians to be willing to explore imaginative possibilities in ways not required of those who do not share the narratives and practices that both make us Christian and, concomitantly, shape our view of the world. Of course, stating the matter in this way is dangerous, for it easily can be interpreted to mean that Christians refuse to acknowledge the world as it "really is." In other words, we open ourselves to the charge that by failing to live in the world "as it really is," our view of the world remains "fantastic" that is, that it arises out of fantasy or illusion.

Yet Christians hold that the so-called world-as-it-really-is is itself fantastic, and so we must learn to live imaginatively, seeing what is not *easily* seen, if we are to faithfully embody the character of the God we worship. Christians are well-aware of how easy it is to live as if the world had no creator. In short, it is easy to live as if we, as well as "nature," had no purpose other than survival. But to live in such a way is not to live in the world "as it is." For to live in the world "as it is" is to be the kind of people who can see that everything has been created to glorify its creator–including the mentally handicapped. To fail to live in such a way is to deny the way the world "is." This is why Christians believe that imagination formed by the storied practices of the church constitutes the ultimate realism.

"Realism" often is used in epistemological contexts to denote that position whose advocates believe objects exist that can be known "in and of themselves." Realists often contrast their views with those who emphasize the importance of the imagination, associating the imagination with fantasy. Imagination is fiction; but knowledge, it is alleged, describes the world "as it is." There is no question that common usage underwrites this kind of distinction between knowledge and imagination–that is, the kind of distinction whose advocates can say, "It's all in her imagination." But as Garret Green observes, it is also the case that people think imagination is essential for helping us know what would otherwise go unnoticed. Thus, we often praise people who demonstrate "insight and imagination" (Green 1989, p. 63).

Much can be said for those like Green who want to rehabilitate imagination as a mode of knowing essential to how Christians think about the world. According to Green, "imagination is the means by which we are able to present anything not directly accessible, including *both* the world of the imaginary *and* recalcitrant aspects of the real world; it is the medium of fiction as well as of fact" (Green 1989, p. 66). Imagination, therefore, seems to be central to the kind of claims that Christians make about God.

However, one problem with proposals like Green's is that such accounts of imagination appear to be too abstract and disembodied. Such accounts accept the assumption that the status of imagination is fundamentally an epistemological issue divorced from the practices of particular communities. On the contrary, however, the Christian imagination is constituted by practices such as non-violence and learning how to be present to–as well as with–the mentally handicapped–who we hopefully know not as mentally handicapped, but as Anna and Boyce, our sister and brother in Christ.

On Children, the Church, and the Mentally Handicapped

Of course, learning to live joyfully with the Annas and the Boyces draws on the resources of other practices that make their presence intelligible in relation to other practices that constitute who we are and desire to be. For example, consider an issue that at first may seem foreign to the question of how we should care for the mentally handicapped–namely, why we have children in the first place. I often used to begin a course in the theology and ethics of marriage with the question: "What reason would you give for yourself or someone else for having a child?" Few students had thought about the question, and their responses were less than convincing: that is, children should manifest their love for one another as a hedge against loneliness, for fun, and/or to please grandparents. Often, one student finally would say that he or she wanted to have children to make the world better. The implicit assumption behind this reason was that the person who spoke up would have superior children who, having received the right kind of training, would be enabled to help solve the world's problems.

Such reasoning often appears morally idealistic. However, its limitations can be revealed quickly by showing its implications for the mentally handicapped. For people who want to have superior children in order to make the world better are deeply threatened by the mentally handicapped. If children are part of a progressive story about the necessity to make the world better, these children do not seem to fit. At best, they only can be understood as deserving existence insofar as our care of them makes us better people.

Such attitudes about having children reveal a society with a deficient moral imagination. It is an imagination correlative to a set of practices about the having and care of children that results in the destruction of the mentally handicapped. The fundamental mistake regarding parenting in our society is the assumption that biology makes parents. In the absences of any good reason for having children, people assume that they have responsibilities to their children because they are biologically "theirs." Lost is any sense of how parenting is an office of a community rather than a biologically described role.

In contrast, Christians assume, given the practice of baptism, that parenting is the vocation of everyone in the church whether they are married or single. Raising children for Christians is part of the church's commitment to hospitality of the stranger, since we believe that the church is sustained by God across generations by witness rather than by ascribed biological destinies. Everyone in the church, therefore, has a parental role whether or not they have biological children.

For Christians, children are neither the entire responsibility nor the property of parents. Parents are given responsibility for particular children insofar as they pledge faithfully to bring up those children, but the community ulti-mately stands over against the parents reminding them that children have a standing in the community separate from their parents. Therefore, the ways in which mentally handicapped children are received in such a community should be strikingly different from how they are received in the wider society. For the whole burden of the care for such children does not fall on the parents; rather, the children now are seen as gifts to the whole community.

At the very least, the church should be the place where parents and mentally handicapped children can be without apologizing, without being stared at, without being silently condemned. If others act as if we ought to be ashamed for having such children among us, then those others will have to take on the whole church. For this is not the child of these biological parents, but this child is the child of the whole church, one whom the church would not choose to be without. Moreover, as this child grows to be an adult, she, just as we all do, is expected to care as well as to be cared for as a member of the church. Such a child may add special burdens to the community but on the average not more than any child. For every child, mentally handicapped or not, always comes to this community challenging our presuppositions. Some children just chal-lenge us more than others as they reveal the limits of our practices. Christians are people who rejoice when we receive such challenges, for we know them to be the source of our imaginations through which God provides us with the skills to have children in a dangerous world. The church is constituted by a people who have been surprised by God and accordingly know that we live through such surprises.

The church, therefore, is that group of people who are willing to have their imagination constantly challenged through the necessities created by children, some of whom may be mentally handicapped. The church is constituted by those people who can take the time in a world crying with injustice to have children, some of whom may turn out to be mentally handicapped. We can do that because we believe this is the way God would rule this world. For we do not believe that the world can be made better if such children are left behind.

I am aware that this view of the church's treatment of the mentally handi-capped is overly idealized. But I believe I am indicating the potential contained in common Christian practice. Moreover, the presence of the mentally handi-capped helps Christians rediscover the significance of the common, because the handicapped call into question some of our most cherished assumptions about what constitutes Christianity. For example, often in Christian communities a great emphasis is placed on the importance of "belief." In attempts to respond to critiques of Christian theology in modernity, the importance of intellectual com-mitments often is taken to be the hallmark of participation in the church. What it means to be Christian is equivalent to being "ultimately concerned" about the existential challenges of human existence and so on. Yet the more emphasis that is placed on belief, particularly for individuals, the more the mentally handicapped are marginalized. For what the mentally handicapped challenge the church to remember is that what saves is not our personal existential commitments, but being a member of a body constituted by practices more determinative than my "personal" commitment. I suspect this is the reason why mentally handicapped people often are better-received in more "liturgical" traditions–that is, traditions which know that what God is doing through the community's ritual is more determinative than what any worshiper brings to or receives from the ritual. After all, the God worshiped is the Spirit that cannot be subject to human control. The liturgy of the church is ordered to be open to such wildness by its hospitality to that Spirit. What the mentally handicapped might do to intrude onto that order is nothing compared to what the Spirit has done and will continue to do. Indeed, the presence of the mentally handicapped may well be the embodiment of the Spirit.

Nowhere is the individualistic and rationalistic character of modern Christianity better revealed than in the practice of Christian education. For example, religious education is often the attempt to "teach" people the content of the Christian faith separate from any determinative practices. What it means to be Christian is to understand this or that doctrine. Yet if the church is the community that is constituted by the presence of the mentally handicapped, we know that salvation cannot be knowing this or that but rather by participating in a community through which our lives are constituted by a unity more profound than our individual needs. From such a perspective the mentally handicapped are not accidental to what the church is about, but without their presence the church has no way to know it is church–that the church is body. If the word is preached and the sacraments served without the presence of the mentally handicapped, then it may be that we are less than the body of Christ.

Mentally handicapped people are reminders that belief and faith are not individual matters, but faith names the stance of the church as a political body in relation to the world. We are not members of a church because we know what we believe, but we are members of a church because we need the whole church to believe for us. Often, if not most of the time, I find that I come to be part of the community that worships God not as a believer or as a faithful follower of Christ, but as someone who is just "not there." I may not be a disbeliever, but I am by no means a believer either. By being present to others in church I find that I am made more than I would otherwise be–I am made one in the faith of the church; my body is constituted by the body called church.

The mentally handicapped remind us that their condition is the condition of us all insofar as we are faithful followers of Christ. The church is not a collection of individuals, but a people on journey who are known by the time they take to help one another along the way. The mentally handicapped constitute such time, as we know that God would not have us try to make the world better if such efforts mean leaving them behind. They are the way we must learn to walk in the journey that God has given us called Kingdom. They are God's imagination, and to the extent we become one with them, we become God's imagination for the world.

Of course, worshipping with the mentally handicapped can be no easy matter. Such worship can be disorderly, since we are never sure what they may or may not do. They create a "wildness" that frightens because they are not easily domesticated. Yet exactly to the extent that they create the unexpected, they remind us that the God we worship is not easily domesticated. For, in worship, the church is made vulnerable to a God that would rule this world not by coercion but through the unpredictability of love. Christians thus learn that the mentally handicapped are not among us because we need someone to be the object of charity, but because without these brothers and sisters in Christ whom we call retarded, we cannot know what it rightly means to worship God.

So through the prism of worship, Christians discover the mentally handicapped as brothers and sisters in Christ. They are not seen as victims of our society. For the great strength of the mentally handicapped is their refusal to be victimized by the temptations to become victims. Through their willingness to be present in church, they provide the church with the time to be the church. We thus learn that we can take the time for someone who does not talk well to read the Scriptures. We can take the time to walk slowly together to the communion table when one of our own does not walk well or not at all. We can take the time to design our places of gathering so that they are open to many who would otherwise not be able to be there. We can take the time to be a people open to children who always will distract us from the projects that seem so promising for making the world "better."

A community formed imaginatively by the presence of the mentally handicapped should, however, provide ways to respond to the challenges and roadblocks mentioned earlier. For if the wider society lacks the basis for knowing how to care for the mentally handicapped, it does so because it is devoid of examples to help it spur its imagination.

What we need to exhibit is that it is not simply the question of how to "care" for the mentally handicapped, but how to be with the mentally handicapped in a way that we learn from them. What any community needs to learn is that the mentally handicapped are not among us to be helped, though like all of us they will need help, but rather by their being among us we learn how we are all more able to be a community. It is interesting, for example, how quickly communities forget how certain practices designed for the "handicapped" become accepted as ways of life for everyone. Thus, a study at the University of Kansas asked why slopes had been put into sidewalks. Most respondents said that they thought that they were there to make bicycling easier. So the access for the handicapped becomes an opportunity for the whole community.

Certainly the ignorance and cruelty of the wider society toward the mentally handicapped needs to be constantly challenged. But more important is the witness of those who have learned that it is not simply a matter of caring for the mentally handicapped but of learning to be with the mentally handicapped. Only when we learn how to be with those different from us can we learn to accept the love that each of us needs to sustain a community capable of worshiping God. It should not be surprising, therefore, that Christians may well be seen in the future as a people who have learned how to be with the mentally handicapped. We may accordingly be thought very odd indeed if our society continues in the direction of the threats discussed above. Yet we believe that nothing could be more significant for a world that assumes that God has not given us the timeful imaginations to be with the mentally handicapped.

Response:
The Limits of Our Practices

Jeff McNair, PhD

SUMMARY. Responding to Professor Hauerwas' essay: "The Church and The Mentally Handicapped," this paper interacts with several of the points made. Specifically, the notion of Christian community, justification for the existence of persons with disability, and Christian imagination. Christians are exhorted in general terms to be more responsive to individuals with disabilities in their midst. *[Article copies available for a fee from The Haworth Document Delivery Service: 1-800-HAWORTH. E-mail address: <docdelivery@haworthpress.com> Website: <http://www.HaworthPress.com> © 2004 by The Haworth Press, Inc. All rights reserved.]*

KEYWORDS. Hauerwas, Christian imagination, disability, churches and disability, church's response to disability

To his credit, Dr. Hauerwas is an individual with an intimate knowledge of and significant experience with individuals with disabilities. His involvement is worthy of note and emulation. His article, *"The Church and the Mentally Handicapped: A Continuing Challenge to the Imagination,"* has obviously

Jeff McNair, is Professor of Special Education/Moderate to Severe Disabilities at California State University, San Bernardino. His program of research relates to the development of community supports for individuals with disability. Specifically, he has studied the role of faith groups. His perspective is informed by over 25 years of Christian ministry to adults with mental retardation.

[Haworth co-indexing entry note]: "Response: The Limits of Our Practices." McNair, Jeff. Co-published simultaneously in *Journal of Religion, Disability & Health* (The Haworth Pastoral Press, an imprint of The Haworth Press, Inc.) Vol. 8, No. 3/4, 2004, pp. 63-69; and: *Critical Reflections on Stanley Hauerwas' Theology of Disability: Disabling Society, Enabling Theology* (ed: John Swinton) The Haworth Pastoral Press, an imprint of The Haworth Press, Inc., 2004, pp. 63-69. Single or multiple copies of this article are available for a fee from The Haworth Document Delivery Service [1-800-HAWORTH, 9:00 a.m. - 5:00 p.m. (EST). E-mail address: docdelivery@haworthpress.com].

grown not only out of his theological reflection, but also his real life experiences. However, I believe Dr. Hauerwas is too kind, and insufficiently confrontational. He would perhaps chuckle at such a characterization.

I would like to respond to Dr. Hauerwas' article on three fronts. First, briefly in relation to his section entitled, *"The 'Problem' of the 'Problem.'"* Then I will respond in more depth to the sections entitled *"The Mentally Handicapped and Christian Imagination,"* and the *"Church and the Mentally Handicapped."* Quotes from Dr. Hauerwas' article are in italics.

THE PROBLEM OF "THE PROBLEM"

The worth of a person is based upon God's valuation of her, and no other arguments on her behalf are required. Of course we should speak up to thwart evil, when we are able. However, if I or anyone else for that matter, is not knowledgeable about someone's purpose, that does not mean he doesn't have a purpose. A preoccupation with the justification argument itself, causes us to look in the wrong direction, to look for a purpose to which no one may be privy. Why is it important to develop arguments to justify the existence of individuals with developmental disabilities to those who would at best ignore and disrespect them, or at worst abort or euthanize them? Even if I were able to convince the detractors, I wonder what they would learn or believe as a result of my efforts, that they didn't know before?

People generally do not feel the need to justify their own existence, as in their own minds they obviously have worth. Those who feel they have no worth are considered mentally ill. We will always enter into arguments over the worth of others at somewhat of a disadvantage. It's not that an argument cannot be made, it's just as the old saying goes, "you can't argue with a sick mind," be it sick due to disease or sick due to prejudice. No rational mind would see only himself or those like himself as having worth.

I personally, have a particularly positive inclination toward persons with disabilities. However, after some 25 plus years of experience in special education and in ministry to adults with developmental disabilities, I have only recently come to the realization that persons with developmental disabilities are simply people trying to live their lives. They are people like me. They have jobs, they live in their homes, they go to the grocery store. They live beyond their means, and think themselves more capable than they are. They choose to do wrong when they know the right thing to do, and they sometimes surprise themselves when they get life right. Those who are religious, worship God to the best of their understanding; meager as such knowledge is in comparison to what might be known. They are simply people like me.

But because of "*the limits of our practices,*" the Church has a limited understanding of who persons with disabilities are. We may even inwardly resonate with attacks of those who would destroy the disabled because on some level, we agree with them. Then in guilt (and partly to convince ourselves), we turn to renewed attempts to justify their existence.

The Mentally Handicapped and Christian Imagination

Imagination is not required to do what might already be done or what is already occurring. It is arguable that Christian imagination is what is keeping the church from acting responsibly toward persons with disabilities. The church rejects, fears, or is disinterested in who they imagine persons with mental retardation to be. They imagine them children, not adults. They are unwanted, but we have to take them. Or as a pastor I know once chided me, "They are a black hole when it comes to service." Christians imagine some service requirement beyond their ability. They imagine how disrupted their lives will become if they take an interest.

Dr. Hauerwas states that "*these examples challenge our imagination concerning how we are to act with the mentally handicapped.*" However, if I imagine a false notion of who disabled individuals are, then I will imagine responses which are probably just as much in error as my original imagined notion. Additionally, Christian imagination need not be about responses yet to be discovered. Clearly over the centuries, Christians have often led the way in imagining innovative, humane ways to treat all types of disenfranchised individuals, and although that is important, it is not generally what is required. Rather, one need only imagine himself doing something, even the most basic thing, and then doing it. Our imaginations need not be stretched to do the incredible, they need to be acted upon to do the simple.

It is interesting to reflect on what it means to be disabled. If someone lives on her own, has a job, enjoys her life, is she disabled? There is little point in characterizing such a person as disabled unless it is necessary in order to receive some particular governmental services. In the United States, with some state agencies, if a disabled individual who is a client is able to find work and no longer needs services from the agency, the agency characterizes that person as having "medically recovered" from his or her disability. That is, one recovers from one's disability through a minimizing of the state supports that are required for an individual to maintain his or her job. In reality, what has probably happened is that the employer or those in the employment environment stepped up to the plate to provide the types of supports the agency would typically provide because they are the types of supports that all employees benefit from to a greater or lesser extent. Using the agency's definition, the Church holds great promise as an agent in the "medical recovery" of individuals with disabilities through the supports it might provide. These supports are of a generic variety, typically provided to a greater or lesser extent to all of the church's members to facilitate their integration into the congregation and the larger community.

Church and the Mentally Handicapped

In his book *The Peaceable Kingdom*, Dr. Hauerwas states that, " . . . we learn to describe by appropriating the narratives of the communities in which we find ourselves" (Hauerwas 1986). It is quite interesting to see the degree to which the Biblical narratives regarding persons with disabilities have *not* been appropriated in determining the types of interactions we might have with persons with disabilities. No doubt the New Testament writers devoted significant time to the miracles of Jesus to support his claims regarding himself, however, one can hardly read a gospel passage without an allusion to a disabled person interacting with Jesus. In one of the most telling passages, Matthew 12, Jesus' enemies need only have an individual with a disabled hand in the audience to "trip him up." Jesus' enemies knew he would see the disabled person and ultimately heal him (on the Sabbath). Obviously this entire interaction was in no way so simple, yet, how interesting it is as an insight into Jesus' awareness of individuals with disabilities. One must wonder why this and other narratives, so ubiquitous in the gospels, have not resulted in more universal changes in church behavior.

In contrast, our responses to individuals with disabilities are to argue about whether a ramp is absolutely required, or whether it "is really that important that the disabled teenager be a member of the youth group, because as you know it has always met on the second floor," or to complain about the inconvenience the autistic child causes in the Sunday School class (actual arguments). My own church recently held a servant celebration to rejoice in congregational members' service. How telling that two mentally handicapped servants sat by themselves off in a corner at a meeting of the church's brightest servants. I suspect there were some who wished they weren't there at all.

We find it easy to confront the world about their disturbing solutions to the *"problem of mental retardation,"* however, it is unfortunate that we can only see the splinter in our neighbor's eye. Even Dr. Hauerwas interrupts his limply radical description of a form of responsibility toward individuals with disabilities with the admission, *"I am aware that this view of the church's treatment of the mentally handicapped is overly idealized."* He attempts to recover from this admission by exhorting, But I believe I am indicating the potential contained in common Christian practice. Moreover, the presence of the mentally handicapped helps Christians rediscover the significance of the common, because the handicapped call into question some of our most cherished assumptions about what constitutes Christianity.

This is once again a justification for existence aimed at detractors, only this time those in the Church. Had this statement been made about just about anyone not suffering disenfranchisement, it might be considered a compliment. However, the same statement in reference to individuals with disability elicits the skeptical glance of mistrust or worry. "Why is it important that I have something to offer you?" "Why must you be able to gain something from me, for me to have value in your eyes?" "Am I in danger if I come to you with nothing but myself?"

Indeed. Christian interactions with individuals with disability are too often more reflective of the negative examples of religious and secular interactions then they are of some God inspired interaction. Many programs that do attempt to serve individuals with disabilities, do so through an approach evidencing a lazy ethic of glassy eyed pity. To individuals who work with the disabled, the constant refrain about the patience it takes to engage in such work, or the excuses offered to veil clandestine discrimination are repeated to the point of being trite. If the disabled do indeed have worth, this should be evident in our religious practice.

Do we prove someone's worth by serving him? To some degree, the answer is yes. His imposed inconvenience tests our commitment. As Dr. Hauerwas points out, it stretches our imagination. But rain engages my imagination to find ways to avoid getting wet, and the answer is not to simply rejoice as I stand out in the midst of it. As Dr. Hauerwas' friend John Yoder described, we bear the cross by what we do to engage others and perhaps challenge their imaginations (Yoder, 1999).

But let's follow this path of existence justification, through challenged imagination. What are we hoping our minds will imagine that will justify the existence of individuals with disability? Professor Hauerwas himself provides the answer. Christian imagination is constituted by practices such as nonviolence and learning to be present to–as well as with–the mentally handicapped, who we hopefully know not as mentally handicapped, but as Anna and Boyce, our sister and brother in Christ.

Our best and brightest hope is to see people with disabilities as no different than ourselves. Once that happens, we will try to do unto them as we would have them do unto us. We must remember that we ourselves are not "a day at the beach." In fact, Jesus felt the need to use his own life to prove our own worth to us.

Dr. Hauerwas says that he doesn't particularly like the term normal. But then, he is a professing Texan. But it is a perfectly fine term, and as Dr. Wolf

Wolfensberger, arguably the one who coined the term "normalization" has said, disabled individuals should simply be treated as normally as possible. They should be respected, loved, or gotten angry at in the same way as any other person. We shed labels and know people.

Ultimately, individuals with disabilities should be integrated into the community as if their disability were as irrelevant a characteristic as hair color or state of origin. Community integration is the critical issue. Christians have the potential to act as mediators between all types of disenfranchised individuals and the groups with whom integration is needed. The community may be resistive, but sometimes the behavioral repertoire of a community needs to be changed. The ideas which originally informed the "that's the way we always have done it" behaviors are outdated and intolerant. Defensiveness within the Christian community will not stretch the community's imagination.

However, with even the slightest level of awareness, we become confronted by "the limits of our practices." Dr. Hauerwas feels we need our imaginations challenged. What has gone wrong is not that we lack goodwill, but that we simply do not know how to care because we need the challenge of real people who teach us how to care. Such people really are the imagination of a community, for we must remember that imagination is not something we have in our minds."

Perhaps he is correct that we actually do not know how to care, or perhaps more likely we are too lazy to find out how to care. An important problem with the church today is the over emphasis on professionalism and excellence. We don't or can't care, because we don't have any training, or we assume that somewhere there is a professional who is being paid to care. In other words, it might often be that we *do* lack goodwill.

Matthew 25 is a passage that speaks directly to our responsibility to care for our neighbor. However, Matthew 25 does not state "that those of you with training who did for one of the least of these my brothers did it unto me." The addition of training or experience is a world imposed standard we as the Church have foolishly embraced. Arguably, we have embraced the idea because it allows us to act irresponsibly toward our neighbor. It isn't that we deliberately seek to harm, but rather that we are not sufficiently interested to care. Interestingly, the presence or absence of a helping interest in others provides an indication to those who are watching us, those who are not yet believers, about how they might expect us to act toward them.

Our practices relative to individuals with disabilities, also tell the world about who we believe God is. "*Imagination is a pointer to a community's constant willingness to expose itself to the innovations required by its convictions about who God is.*" What do we imagine our practices are telling the secular community, about who God is? How wonderful if observers looked on the church and learned that God is not a labeler, for example, who characterizes people by a supposedly logical notion of mental age. That God is not one who will pass the buck to state agent professionals, but is a servant who steps up to meet even the most difficult of challenges because he wants to be a servant. That God is one who accepts all persons, independent of personal characteristics. That God does not evaluate a person on the basis of the contribution he can make. That God proves the worth of a person once and for all through Jesus giving his life for people who could not save themselves.

CONCLUSION

Christians have to want persons with disabilities in their homes and in their lives. The names of disabled congregational members should be known to their children. Not because of some syrupy sentimental notion that their children will gain something (though they may), or that the disabled members will in some way justify their existence through their presence, their words or their actions. Rather, it is because individuals with disabilities are people worth getting to know. People with disabilities are not that different from persons without disabilities. The Church of Jesus Christ above all needs to learn this, and then perhaps as Dr. Hauerwas dreams, *"be seen in the future as a people who have learned how to be with the mentally handicapped."* I pray for that day. Christians must out human the humanists.

REFERENCES

Hauerwas, Stanley (1986). *The Peaceable Kingdom.* Notre Dame, Indiana: University of Notre Dame Press.

Yoder, John Howard (1999). *The Politics of Jesus.* Grand Rapids, Michigan: Eerdmans.

Chapter 4

The Gesture of a Truthful Story

Stanley Hauerwas, PhD

[From *Theology Today*-Volume 42, No 2-July 1985, pp. 181-189.] Reprinted with permission.

SUMMARY. Hauerwas presents a moral vision of the church and reframes the way in which we might understand Christian education. He presents a model of the church *as* a social ethic. The church does not simply *do* ethics, it *is* an ethic insofar as it embodies the gestures of the coming Kingdom and reveals the good-life that is found in Christ. Hauerwas argues that religious education is the training in those gestures through which we learn the story, of God and God's will for our lives . . . It is ongoing training in the skills we need in order to live faithful to the kingdom that has been initiated in Jesus. Hauerwas suggests that the 'mentally handicapped' are a reminder, a test case, for helping us understand how any account of religious education involves assumptions about the nature of Christian conviction and the church. It is certainly true that they may not be able to read the story; nor are they always able to "understand" the "meaning" of the story nor do they know what social implications the

---

[Haworth co-indexing entry note]: "The Gesture of a Truthful Story." Hauerwas, Stanley. Co-published simultaneously in *Journal of Religion, Disability & Health* (The Haworth Pastoral Press, an imprint of The Haworth Press, Inc.) Vol. 8, No. 3/4, 2004, pp. 71-80; and: *Critical Reflections on Stanley Hauerwas' Theology of Disability: Disabling Society, Enabling Theology* (ed: John Swinton) The Haworth Pastoral Press, an imprint of The Haworth Press, Inc., 2004, pp. 71-80. Single or multiple copies of this article are available for a fee from The Haworth Document Delivery Service [1-800-HAWORTH, 9:00 a.m. - 5:00 p.m. (EST). E-mail address: docdelivery@haworthpress.com].

story may entail. But what they do know is who the story is embodied through the essential gestures of the church. They know the story through the care they receive, and they help the church understand the story that forms such care.

KEYWORDS. Education, story, gestures, community, exemplars

It is ongoing training in the skills we need in order to live faithful to the kingdom that has been initiated in Jesus. "I worry about the idea that religious education is some special activity separated from the total life of the church. When that happens, it makes it appear that what the church does in its worship is something different from what it does in its education. I would contend that everything the church is and does is "religious education." Put more strongly, the church does not "do" religious education at all. Rather, the church *is* a form of education that is religious. Moreover, if that is the case, then I think there is a very close relation between Christian education and social ethics–at least if how I understand social ethics is close to being right. Such an assertion is by no means clear, nor is its implications immediately apparent. I will try to unravel that claim by analyzing first a similar contention about Christian social ethics–namely, that the church does not have a social ethic, but rather is a social ethic.

The claim that the church is a social ethic is an attempt to remind us that the church is the place where the story of God is enacted, told, and heard. Christian social ethics is not first of all principles or policies for social action, but rather the story of God's calling of Israel and of the life of Jesus. That story requires the formation of a corresponding community that has learned to live in ways appropriate to them. The church does not have a social ethic, but is a social ethic, then, insofar as it is a community that can clearly be distinguished from the world. For the world is not a community and has no such story, since it is based on the assumption that human beings, not God, rule history. Therefore, the first social task of the church is to help the world know that it is the world. For without the church, the world has no means to know that it is the world. The distinction between church and the world is not a distinction between nature and grace. It is, instead, a distinction that denotes "the basic personal postures of men, some of who confess and others of whom do not confess that Jesus Christ is Lord. The distinction between church and the world is not something that God has imposed upon the world by prior metaphysical definition, nor is it only something, which timid or pharisaical Christians have built up around themselves. It is all of that in creation that has taken the freedom not yet to believe."

The fact that the church is separated from the world is not meant to underwrite an ethic of self-righteousness on the part of the church. Both church and world remain under the judgment of the Kingdom of God. Indeed, we must remember that the church is but the earnest of the Kingdom. Those of us who attempt to live faithful to that Kingdom are acutely aware how deeply our lives remain held to and by the world. But this cannot be an excuse for acting as if there is no difference between the world and us. For if we use our sin to deny our peculiar task as Christians and as members of the church, we are unfaithful both to the Kingdom and to ourselves and most importantly to the world itself. Moreover, when we deny the distinctive task of the church, we implicitly deny the particularity of the narrative that makes us what we are in the first place. As Christians, we are not after all called to be morally good, but rather to be faithful to the story that we claim is truthful to the very character of reality which is that we are creatures of a gracious God who asks nothing less of us than faithful service to God's Kingdom. In short, we are people who know who is in control. What it means to be Christian, therefore, is that we are a people who affirm that we have come to find our true destiny only by locating our lives within the story of God. The church is the lively argument, extended over centuries and occasioned by the stories of God's calling of Israel and of the life and death of Jesus Christ, to which we are invited to contribute by learning to live faithful to those stories. It is the astounding claim of Christians that through this particular man's story, we discover our true selves and thus are made part of God's very life. We become part of God's story by finding our lives within that story. For the church to be, rather than to have, a social ethic means that it must be a community where the truth is lived and spoken.

The story that forms the church is as I have suggested, a reality-making claim that tells us the truth about the world and ourselves. Such truth is indeed hard. It means that we cannot know the truth until we have been transformed by the story. We cannot know Jesus without becoming his disciples. There is, therefore, an unavoidably self-involving character to Christian convictions. It requires that our very selves be transformed if we are to face the truth that we are sinners yet saved. A community of such people cannot help but be a social ethic, since it must stand in sharp contrast with the world, which would have us, build our relations on distortions and denials. The world is where the truth is not spoken for fear such truth might destroy what fragile order and justice we behave been able to achieve. But the church, which claims to be construed by a people who have no fear of the truth, must be a polity where the truth is spoken, even if such truth risks pain and threatens disorder. The church is thus a polity that takes as its constitution a story whose truth creates a people who love honestly, because they have the confidence that such love binds our lives to God's very character.

Such a community cannot help but stand in sharp contrast with the world. A people formed in the likeness of God cannot be anything less than a community of character. That is, it is a community which takes as its task the initiation of people into the story in a manner that forms and shapes their lives in a decisive and distinctive way. Put bluntly, the church is in the world to mark us. The church, therefore, alms not at autonomy, but at faithfulness. We believe that it is only as we learn to be faithful that we have the ability to be free. Freedom, contrary to much contemporary thought, consists not in having no story, but rather comes only through being trained and acquiring the skills of a truthful story.

That is why the church, in contrast to many communities, knows that the only way to learn to be faithful is through initiation by a master. Most of contemporary morality, both in its philosophical and popular expression assumes that the moral life is an achievement that is open to anyone. On such a view of the moral life, what is required is not a master, but simply the ability to make well-reasoned decisions. In contrast, the church knows that the life of faithfulness is not easily acquired, but involves those skills that can be learned only through apprenticeship to a master. Living morally is not simply holding the right principles; it involves nothing less than learning to desire the right things rightly. Such desiring is not so much a matter or choice as it is the slow training of our vision through learning to pay attention to the insignificant. Such attention is gained only as we have the story mediated to us by masters who have learned what the story says by learning how, difficult it is to hear it. In short, the church, Christians, are the group of people capable of engendering and recognizing saints. To be able to do that is no small feat. Saints cannot exist without a community, as they require, like all of us, nurturance by a people who, while often unfaithful, preserve the habits necessary to learn the story of God. Moreover, such a community must have the skills of discernment that make them capable of recognizing the saints in their midst. Recognizing the saints, especially while they are still alive, is no easy task either. For by their very nature, saints remind us how unfaithful we have been to the story that has formed us.

To be a community capable of engendering as well as of recognizing the saints requires that we be a people formed by the virtues of hope and patience. These are the virtues, the habits, crucial to learning well the story of God. To learn that story means we must desire nothing less than the accomplishment of God's rule, the Kingdom, over all nations and peoples. That rule is nothing less than the establishment of peace between ourselves and God, from which we learn how to be peaceful in ourselves and with one another. Because we have tasted this peace, because we have found how marvelous it is to have violence rooted out of our souls, is why we so desperately desire it for all. We know, God's peace is not easily made one's own. But we have confidence that if we are faithful to God's Kingdom, God will use our faithfulness to realize this Kingdom for all. But just to the extent that we have been taught to hope, we must also be patient. For God does not will that the Kingdom be accomplished through coercion or violence. In the cross, we see how the Kingdom will come into the world, and we are charged to be nothing less than a cruciform people. We must, then, learn to wait as we seek to manifest to the world God's peace that comes into our lives by no other means than the power of that truth itself. Such waiting is painful indeed in a world as unjust and violent as ours. But we believe it justified, since we have been promised that God will use our waiting for the complete triumph of the Kingdom.

Moreover, patience is required because at least part of what it means for the church to be, rather than to have, a social ethic involves a rethinking about what is meant by social ethics. Too often, in an effort to appear socially relevant, the church has accepted the world's agenda about what "real" politics involves. Thus, calls for us to serve the world responsibly have too often resulted in the church simply saying to the world what the world already knows. We thereby end up trying to secure a "justice" which is only the continuation of some people's domination of others. In contrast, I am suggesting we must be a patient people, as well as a courageous people, who have the skills to think through the current illusions about social justice and peace. We must be the kind of community that can draw on the character of convictions that expose the sentimentalities or the world–not the least of which is the assumption that nation-states have the right to qualify our loyalty as members of the church. It takes a patient as well as courageous people to manifest that the unity of God's eschatological meal is the only true internationalism.

Such a meal:

> posits and proclaims a unification of mankind whose basis is not some as yet unachieved restructuring of political sovereignties but an already achieved transformation of vision and community. That all mankind is one cannot be demonstrated empirically nor can political engineering bring it about. That all mankind is one must first be affirmed as a theological proclamation. Only then is the engineering and structuring which are needed to reflect it even conceivable. It could just as well be said that Christian internationalism is the true unity which the servant church must let be restored. (Yoder 1977, p. 130)

Nor must we forget that the most embarrassing divisions in the church are not between Catholic and Protestant, U.C.C. and Methodist, Presbyterian and Church of Christ, liberal and conservative, but between social and economic class, race, and nationalities. Such divisions give lie to the fact that we are one people rooted in the God who has called us into the Kingdom inaugurated by Jesus' life and death. Thus, the first concern of any Christian social ethic must be with the fellowship of the church. We must be a community with the patience, amid the division and hatreds of this world, to take the time to nurture friendships, to serve the neighbor, and to give and receive the thousand small acts of care that ultimately are the heart blood of the Kingdom. That we must take the time to help the neighbor in need, no matter how insignificant that neighbor or his or her need is from the perspective of the world, is but a sign that we recognize that we are called not to make history come out right, but to be faithful to the kind of care we have seen revealed in God's Kingdom. In this respect, the church as a social ethic must take its lead from those like Mother Teresa. From a perspective that would associate the church's social task with effectiveness, Mother Teresa is a deeply immoral woman. She takes the time to hold the hand of a dying leprosy victim when she could be raising money in Europe and America for the starving in India. Yet, she sits there holding the hand of a dying person–doing that while surrounded by unbelievable suffering and injustice–because she knows that God will have the Kingdom come exactly by such care. And she knows she can do so because she does not seek to be like the powerful to help the poor and dying. She has learned instead that power derives from being faithful to God's Kingdom of the poor.

This, surely, is not the word we want to hear today. We want a word that puts the church on the right side for a change–the side for political change and justice. This news I bring, therefore, seems more bad than good. If being Christian does not put us where the action is, if being Christian does not put us on the side of the progressive forces in this or any other society, then I suspect many of us would be a good deal less happy with being Christian. The claim that the church is, rather than has, a social ethic cannot help but appear to many as a dangerous withdrawal of the church back into a self-righteous pietism that ignores the social agony of the world. At best, such a Christian social ethic is but a gesture; at worst, it is a failure of Christians to face responsibly the complexity of the social problems confronting us in these troubled times.

I am ready to concede that the church, and Christian social ethics, as I have tried to depict it, is but a gesture, but I do not think that to be a damaging admission. For nothing in life is more important than gestures, as gestures embody as well as sustain the valuable and significant. Through gestures, we create and form our worlds. Through gestures, we make contact with one another and share common tasks. Through gestures, we communicate and learn from each other the limits of our world. In this sense, the church is but God's gesture on behalf of the world to create a space and time in which we might have a foretaste of the Kingdom. It is through gestures that we learn the nature of the story that is the very content and constitution of that Kingdom. The way we learn a story, after all, is not just by hearing it. Important and significant stories must be acted out. We must be taught the gestures that help position our bodies and our souls to be able to rightly hear and then retell the story. For example, while we may be able to pray without being prostrate, I think prayer as an institution of the church could no longer be sustained without a people who have first learned to kneel. If you want to learn to pray, you had better know how to bend the body. The gesture and posture of prayer are inseparable from learning to pray. Indeed, the gestures are prayer.

Of course, some of our most important gestures are words. But we can easily overestimate their significance if we assume that words can be separated from the context of their enactment. For example, the Apostles' Creed is not simply a statement of faith that can stand independent of the context in which we affirm it. We must learn to say it in the context of worship if we are to understand how it works to rule our belief and school our faith. The Creed is not some deposit or sum of the story; rather, it is a series of reminders about how best to tell the story that we find enacted through the entire liturgy. In the same way, baptism and the eucharist stand as crucial gestures that are meant to shape us rightly to hear as well as enact the story. Through baptism and eucharist, we are initiated into God's life by our becoming part of Jesus' life, death, and resurrection. These are essential gestures of the church; we cannot be the church without them. They are, in effect, essential reminders for the constitution of God's people in the world. Without them, we are constantly tempted to turn God into an ideology to supply our wants and needs rather than have our needs and wants transformed by God's capturing of our attention through the mundane life of Jesus of Nazareth.

Thus, liturgy is not a motive for social action, it is not a cause to effect. Liturgy is social action. Through liturgy we are shaped to live rightly the story of God, to become part of that story, and are thus able to recognize and respond to the saints in our midst. Once we recognize that the church is a social ethic, an ethic that is to be sure but a gesture, then we can appreciate how every activity of the church is a means and an opportunity for faithful service to and for the world. We believe that the gesture that is the church is nothing less than the sign of God's salvation of the world. But what does all this have to do with Christian education–and, in particular, the claim that the church does not do religious education, but is a form of education that is religious? First of all, it reminds us that religious education has as its first task the initiation of a people into a story. Its task is not to teach us the meaning of that story, but to teach us the story. There is no point that can be known separate from the story. There is no experience that we want people to have apart from the story. There are no "moral lessons" that we wish to inculcate other than the story. The story is the point, the story is the experience, and the story is the moral.

The task of religious education therefore involves the development of skills to help us make the story ours. Or, perhaps better, the task of religious education is to help remind us of those skills present in the church that are essential for helping us make the story ours. Such reminders may well involve psychological insights about how such skills work, but the former cannot be a substitute for the latter. The content of the story must control where and how the story is to be made our own.

Put simply, religious education is the training in those gestures through which we learn the story of God and God's will for our lives. Religious education is not, therefore, something that is done to make us Christians, or something done after we have become Christian. Rather, it is ongoing training in the skills we need in order to live faithful to the Kingdom that has been initiated in Jesus. That Kingdom is constituted by a story that one never possesses, but rather constantly challenges us to be what we are but have not yet become. The primary task of being educated religiously, or better Christianly, is not the achievement of better understanding but faithfulness. Indeed, we can only come to understand through faithfulness as the story, and the corresponding community, which forms our life, asks nothing less from us than our life. The story requires that we learn to live as a people who have been forgiven and thus can be at peace with ourselves as well as with others. We do not learn to be forgiven by intellectually admitting that we often have failed to live up to our own moral ideals, but rather by learning to depend on God as the source of life and the sustainer of our community. What we are asked to be is first and foremost a people who embody and manifest the habits of peace characteristic of a forgiven people–not just those world who provide worldviews through which to make sense of the world. We become faithful just to the extent that we learn to participate in the activities of the people of God we call the church. Therefore, it becomes our duty to be a people who submit to the discipline of the liturgy, as it is there that we are trained with the skills rightly to know the story. We are required to care for one another, and to accept the care of others, for it is by learning to be cared for that we learn to care. Such duties may be no more than gestures, but they are the essential gestures that initiate us into the narrative of God's dealing with people.

Yet all this may still sound far too abstract. Therefore, let me try to provide a concrete case that I hope will draw out the implications of the position I have tried to develop. One of the tasks people concerned with religious education have taken for themselves has been the attempt to find ways to help people better understand what it means to be a Christian. This most often has naturally taken the form of encouraging greater study of Scripture and theology, the assumption being that we will be better Christians if we simply know more. While I have nothing against the study of Scripture and theology, I think our emphasis in that respect has tended to make us forget that the way we learn the story is by learning such gestures as simple as how to kneel. More troubling, such an emphasis excludes in a decisive manner a whole group of people from participation in God's Kingdom. For what do you do with the mentally handicapped?

The mentally handicapped are a reminder, a test case, for helping us understand how any account of religious education involves assumptions about the nature of Christian conviction and the church. It is certainly true that the mentally handicapped may not be able to read the story; nor are they always able to "understand" the "meaning" of the story nor do they know what the social implications the story may entail. But what they do know is who the story is embodied through the essential gestures of the church. They know the story through the care they receive, and they help the church understand the story that forms such care. Moreover, they learn the story through its enactment as they feel and are formed by the liturgy that places us as characters in God's grand project of the creation and redemption of the world. They know that they too have a role in God's people as they faithfully serve God through being formed by a community that is nothing less than the enactment of that story. It is important that we guard against a possible misunderstanding that may be occasioned by the interjection of the place of the mentally handicapped in religious education. I am not suggesting that the retarded represent some bottom line or minimum that must be met for religious education. On the contrary, I am suggesting that they, and I am sure there are other equally compelling examples, offer a clue about the center of the task of Christian education and why it is that the church as such is Christian education. For if faithfulness is our task, if it is through faithfulness that we rightly learn to hear, tell, and embody the story, then the mentally handicapped are a crucial and ever present reminder that such is the case.

Nor am I suggesting that the mentally handicapped are somehow naturally ready to be formed by the story. They are no fewer sinners than any of the rest of us. Their desires require training no less than our desires. Faithfulness is not a natural task for the mentally handicapped or for us. We equally must be trained to face the world, as it is not as we would like it to be. In like measure, we all must learn to accept and give forgiveness, as we also must learn to be people of peace and justice.

However, there is another connection between the argument I have tried to make about the church as a social ethic, the implications of that for religious education, and the mentally handicapped. For at least part of what it means for the church to be a social ethic is that it has the time to care in an unjust world for those who do not promise to make the world better, more just, or direct the course of history. The church as God's gesture in and for the world must be the people who manifest our conviction that we do not live on the world's time, but in God's time. I suspect we do that best when we show ourselves to be a people who have the time to care for one another even when some of us happen to be mentally handicapped.

It may seem extremely odd to end an essay on Christian education by calling attention to the mentally handicapped. To end there seems to suggest that our intellectual skills are not as important as we would like to think. I must admit, moreover, that I am not entirely unhappy with such a conclusion–even though it is clearly exaggerated. After all, I am among those who have engaged in that most ambiguous enterprise that we identify as theology. And I believe that the church is less if it does not engender and sponsor the critical activity we call theology.

Yet, in an interesting way, that activity, and the educational institution necessary to sustain it, draws on the same presuppostions and virtues that sustains the church's commitment to having the mentally handicapped among us. For the activity of theology can only be sustained by a community that has learned to wait patiently in a world of suffering and injustice. Theology and theologians do little to make the world better. Rather, our craft involves the slow and painful steps of trying to understand better what it means to be a people formed by the story of God. Let us not forget, then, that, as theologians, we no less than the mentally retarded depend on and serve a church which provides us with the gestures necessary to being the people of God.

REFERENCES

Hauerwas, Stanley. (1981). *A Community of Character: Toward a Constructive Christian Social Ethic.* Notre Dame: University of Notre Dame Press.
_____*The Peaceable Kingdom: A Primer in Christian Ethics.* (1983). Notre Dame: University of Notre Dame Press.
John Howard Yoder. (1977). *The Original Revolution.* Scottdale, PA: Herald Press, 1971, p. 116.

Response:
On Discovering Saints
and Making a Difference

Aileen Barclay, PhD (cand.)

SUMMARY. This response expresses reservations about the portrayal of the church as an exclusive institution, concerned more with its own formation than with educational processes which would raise consciousness about how ways in which people can respond to the kingdom in their own contexts. Two main reservations are presented. The first asks questions about the distinctiveness and difference of Christian social ethics while the second questions how the truth of the story that the church tells can be known. The author suggests that education has a broader meaning and application than simply initiation into a story and training in specific skills and that the institutional church would do well to listen to the voices beyond its own walls, particularly in the communities of people living with disabilities. *[Article copies available for a fee from The Haworth Document Delivery Service: 1-800-HAWORTH. E-mail address: <docdelivery@haworthpress.com> Website: <http://www.HaworthPress.com> © 2004 by The Haworth Press, Inc. All rights reserved.]*

Aileen Barclay lectures in Educational Studies at the University of Aberdeen, Scotland, UK. Previously she was an Education Officer with responsibility for Support for Learners and Children's Issues with Aberdeenshire Council. A native of Aberdeen, she taught as a Primary School teacher and then as a teacher of Special Educational Needs in a Secondary School. She is currently working towards a PhD in Practical Theology at the University of Aberdeen.

[Haworth co-indexing entry note]: "Response: On Discovering Saints and Making a Difference." Barclay, Aileen. Co-published simultaneously in *Journal of Religion, Disability & Health* (The Haworth Pastoral Press, an imprint of The Haworth Press, Inc.) Vol. 8, No. 3/4, 2004, pp. 81-85; and: *Critical Reflections on Stanley Hauerwas' Theology of Disability: Disabling Society, Enabling Theology* (ed: John Swinton) The Haworth Pastoral Press, an imprint of The Haworth Press, Inc., 2004, pp. 81-85. Single or multiple copies of this article are available for a fee from The Haworth Document Delivery Service [1-800-HAWORTH, 9:00 a.m. - 5:00 p.m. (EST). E-mail address: docdelivery@haworthpress.com].

http://www.haworthpress.com/web/JRDH
© 2004 by The Haworth Press, Inc. All rights reserved.
Digital Object Identifier: 10.1300/J095v8n03_10

KEYWORDS. Inclusion, social ethics, saints, education, freedom

Having come late to knowledge of the truthful story, I concede that I have still much to learn. Professor Hauerwas' evocative essay has enabled me to reflect on the nature of that story helping me to sharpen my own gestures as I struggle to live out the meaning of being human in a world that is often profoundly dehumanising. For this I am grateful.

THE QUESTION OF INCLUSION

It is clear to me that Professor Hauerwas writes with a sense of deep commitment from a traditional evangelical (with a small e) standpoint. His passion is obvious and his commitment to the gospel as "lived experience" helpfully brings together theory and practice and embodies it in human relationships within community. With that, I identify wholly! Nevertheless, I do have certain reservations about the way in which the church-as-community is portrayed, at least metaphorically, as an exclusive institution. Hauerwas' model of the church seems to me rather inward looking, concerned more with its own formation than with the practical educational processes which are necessary for raising Christian consciousness in such a way that people can respond to the story of the Kingdom in their own contexts. In order to clarify and draw out what I mean by this, I will explore two areas of Hauerwas' thinking that I consider would benefit from further exploration. They are as follows:

- What is distinctive about a Christian social ethic?
- Can we be sure that the story the church tells is the truthful story?

What Is Distinctive About a Christian Social Ethic?

My personal answer to this question is that the distinctiveness of a Christian social ethic lies in the recognition of freedom at a spiritual, personal, and socio-political level. As our 'spirits' are freed, so we can reach beyond the perceived reality towards knowledge of the ultimate Transcendent One. Here we discover moral and existential security and the motivation and drive to live out the gospel. By God's grace we are personally set free to commune with God and others. Of course, in saying this I reveal my liberal roots, as I am certain Professor Hauerwas would be quick to highlight. Surely, he might argue, the essence of the gospel is that we are not free, equal individuals, but that we are "slaves in Christ." Freedom and equality in the way some of our society understands them are illusory, false and ultimately destructive, particularly for people with "mental handicap." He may be right. But I still believe that freedom remains an important Christian concept. Nevertheless, personal and social freedom is difficult to achieve in the face of destructive societal structures and Christians are also called to live in opposition to such structures. My worry about Hauerwas' understanding of church-as-community is that it appears to withdraw from the world, leaving open the possibility of elitism, prejudice, and a lack of responsibility for what goes on in "the real world."

Professor Hauerwas argues that the church is a social ethic rather than has a social ethic (Hauerwas 1981; 1983). This is a strong point. It is only as ethics are embodied in loving gestures that they become ethics in any meaningful sense. However, one is still left with the question: What is the significance of the uniqueness of that ethic?

What Is Different About the Christian Social Ethic?

At the heart of all world religions is a social ethic with potential to benefit all humanity. It seems to me that the distinctive of Christianity lies not simply in the church community or the ethic that emerges from that community. Rather, the distinctive is found in the gift of a vulnerable God who comes to us not just to create a safe enclave within which we can develop our characters and wait out the present tribulation in the hope of salvation in the next life. Rather, this vulnerable God sends us out into the world with the hope that *in the world* through recognition of Jesus as Liberator as well as Redeemer and Saviour, we can participate "in eager expectation . . . that the creation itself will be liberated from its bondage to decay" (Romans 8:19-20 NIV). Within such a process, we meet with God not only in community, but also in our relationships with others, (those who share and those who do not share our ethic) as a forgiven and forgiving people sustained in the faith that God stands in solidarity with us in the whole-of-our-lives-in-the-world. I am not sure that Hauerwas' community could achieve such a goal. Hauerwas refers to those who do not share the Christian narrative as: "all of that in creation that has taken the freedom not yet to believe" (Yoder 1971, p. 116). Of course, as a Christian I understand the significance of faith, belief and commitment to Jesus as Lord and Saviour. However, to think of church and the world in such dichotomous terms sits uneasily with me.

I can't help feeling that the distinction made by Professor Hauerwas between church and world is potentially destructive and open to abuse by the perpetuation of divisiveness and hatred. The life experiences of people in Northern Ireland and the Middle East bear witness to the consequence of religious bigotry. In a post 9/11 world, can we justify such a potentially divisory position?

Hauerwas may well be correct in his emphasis on the significance of ritual for the consolidation and well being of the church community, but again I find myself worrying. My personal experience of institutionalised church would suggest that conformity to liturgy can be a double-edged sword. Certainly it can bring liberation and healing. But it can also be nothing more than an external demonstration of human power, which can be given priority over living the type of spiritual life to which Hauerwas alludes. External demonstrations can also cover up negative states of mind such as anger, hatred and greed, and jealousy. When this happens, liturgy can become a form of social closure rather than a source of liberation, with conformity to ritual bringing a sense of belonging and connection to tradition for some, while at the same time excluding others who are forced to endure liturgy fundamentally disconnected from the reality of struggling, fragmented, and broken lives.

I do not know if the people with whom I have shared much of my life belong to the group Professor Hauerwas refers to as church, and I do not believe that God asks me to make that kind of judgement. However, I do know that by participating as a partner with families affected by disability, poverty, and other forms of oppression, I am learning what it means to be a relational creature made in the image of a vulnerable God and therefore set free by faith to stand in opposition to structures opposed to Kingdom values.

Telling a Truthful Story?

As a professional educator, I have found myself struggling with the distinction Professor Hauerwas makes between education which is specifically religious and other forms of education. I remain uncertain precisely what he means by "religious education." As I reflect on scripture, it is clear that Christian learning takes place in a variety of settings involving observation, participation, listening, discussion, action-reflection, and instruction involving the whole of life. Christian learning does not simply relate to initiation into a story and training in some skills. As an educator, I am more comfortable with the broader perspective that I discover in scripture.

On Discovering Saints

Hauerwas' comments on the nature of saints is interesting. He states that: "Christians, are the group of people capable of engendering and recognising saints. . . . Saints cannot exist without a community, as they require, like all of us, nurturance by a people who, while often unfaithful, preserve the habits necessary to learn the story of God." Hauerwas may be right, but most of the saints that I have encountered in my personal and professional life have no connection with Hauerwas' community. Through observing children and their families, through participating with them in their often painful journeys, through listening to their cries, discussing and reflecting on experience I have been privileged to meet many 'saints' who have had little recognition for the lives they lead but from whom I have learned much. For me, the 'saints' are the wide spectrum of people, including parents and children and young people with disabilities as well as paid professionals who, through their compassionate actions, can be found telling love stories to those in our society who have little voice. The saints not only care for physical and emotional needs, they also ensure that the system knows and responds to the contribution individuals and groups make. In this way they secure opportunities for all to flourish in spite of the gross inequalities of the world in which we live. I have been humbled by the creative ways in which people who are marginalised in school and society have been able to overcome obstacles, which would have a devastating affect on people who enjoy more privileged lifestyles. Perhaps, rather than the Christian community being a witness to these people, it often strikes me just what a prophetic witness such saints are to the church. The question is, does the community of the church listen to and acknowledge the gestures from outside the boundaries?

CONCLUSION

To the Jews who had believed Him, Jesus said, "If you hold to my teaching, you really are my disciples. Then you will know the truth, and the truth will set you free" (John 8:31-32). We are indeed "slaves to Christ" but in that slavery we are set free to search for the truth as He taught us in the contexts in which we live. As co-partners in the gospel we have the freedom to tell a truthful story and to learn Kingdom gestures which will embody and reveal God's love to those who still do not know the truth of the Christian story. I would like to thank Professor Hauerwas for a stimulating discussion and particularly for raising issues, which have challenged me to think more deeply about the theology of disability.

REFERENCE

Ryrie, C. C. (1986). *The Ryrie Study Bible New International Version.* The Moody Bible Institute of Chicago Zondervan Bible Publishers.

Chapter 5

Suffering the Retarded:
Should We Prevent Retardation?

Stanley Hauerwas, PhD

[From *Suffering Presence: Theological Reflections on Medicine, the Mentally Handicapped, and the Church*. 1986, pp. 159-182.] Reprinted with permission.

SUMMARY. In this essay Hauerwas explores the question of suffering. Does developmental disability necessarily have to be equated with suffering? He explores the nature of suffering in its physical, psychological, and social dimensions and relates this understanding to the life situations of people with developmental disabilities. Hauerwas distinguishes different dimensions of suffering and makes a case for suggesting that suffering when applied to the lives of people with developmental disabilities takes on a deeper and more social meaning. The suffering they experience may well be more extrinsic than intrinsic to their particular condition. Reflect-

Much in the closing paragraph the author has learned from Rev. James Burtchaell. The author would like to thank Mr. Phil Foubert, Rev. Paul Wadell, and Dr. Bonita Raine for reading and criticizing an earlier draft of this article and making valuable suggestions for its improvement.

[Haworth co-indexing entry note]: "Suffering the Retarded: Should We Prevent Retardation?". Hauerwas, Stanley. Co-published simultaneously in *Journal of Religion, Disability & Health* (The Haworth Pastoral Press, an imprint of The Haworth Press, Inc.) Vol. 8, No. 3/4, 2004, pp. 87-106; and: *Critical Reflections on Stanley Hauerwas' Theology of Disability: Disabling Society, Enabling Theology* (ed: John Swinton) The Haworth Pastoral Press, an imprint of The Haworth Press, Inc., 2004, pp. 87-106. Single or multiple copies of this article are available for a fee from The Haworth Document Delivery Service [1-800-HAWORTH, 9:00 a.m. - 5:00 p.m. (EST). E-mail address: docdelivery@haworthpress.com].

http://www.haworthpress.com/web/JRDH
Digital Object Identifier: 10.1300/J095v8n03_11

ing on the theology of Arthur McGill, Hauerwas presents a model of understanding developmental disabilities within the framework of the body of Christ. If the face of God is found in the face of "the retarded," what does that tell us about the nature and purposes of our communities?

KEYWORDS. Suffering, disability, Arthur McGill

A SHORT MOVIE AND A QUESTION

The movie begins. A man and woman looking into a baby crib. The baby is never shown. The room is dark and the countenance of the couple is yet darker. They have obviously been through a trauma and are still in shock. The joy and excitement associated with the birth of a child has been crushed from their lives. Their high expectations have been transformed to absolute despair. They turn toward us and the man speaks: "Don't let this happen to you. Our child was born retarded. He will never play the way other children play. He will not be able to go to school with other children. He will never have an independent existence and will require us to care for him throughout his and our lifetime. Our lives have been ruined. It is too late for us but not for you."

The mother speaks: "Don't let what happened to us happen to you. Be tested early if you think you are pregnant. Maintain good prenatal care under the direction of a physician. Do not smoke, drink, or take any drugs except those absolutely necessary for your health. Please do not let this happen to you–prevent retardation."

A film very much like this was sponsored a few years ago by the American Association of Retarded Citizens. No doubt the film was made with the best of intentions and concern. Surely we ought to prevent retardation. Certainly as many couples as can ought to be encouraged to maintain good prenatal care. Moreover the Association of Retarded Citizens is probably right to assume they will stand a better chance of getting research funds for the retarded if they can convince the public, and thus the government, that their long-term policy is to eliminate retardation like cancer. For if retardation can be eliminated, then the amount of moneys needed for constant care will be significantly reduced. Better a short-term outlay now than a continuing cost.

Nevertheless there seems to be something deeply wrong, something disturbing about this film and its message, "Prevent Retardation." Perhaps, part of the difficulty involves the analogy between preventing retardation and preventing cancer, polio, or heart disease, as these latter diseases exist independent of the subjects having diseases. The disease can be eliminated without eliminating the subject of the disease. But the same is not always true of the retarded. To eliminate retardation may sometimes mean to eliminate the subject. Yet surely this point is not decisive. The film, after all, is not suggesting that we kill anyone who is presently retarded. On the contrary, those who produced the film have dedicated their lives to enhancing the lives of retarded citizens. They have led the war on unjust forms of discrimination against retarded people. They surely do not seek to make the lot of the retarded worse than it is already, rather they simply seek to prevent some from being born unnecessarily retarded. What could be wrong with that?

Still I think something is wrong with a general policy that seeks to prevent retardation, but to say what is wrong with such a policy, involves some of the most profound questions of human existence, including our relationship to God. In particular, assumptions about the nature and necessity of suffering, and our willingness to endure it in our own and other's lives, will need to be addressed. For the very humanity that causes us to cry out against suffering, that motivates us to seek to eliminate retardation, is also the source of our potentially greatest inhumanity. By trying to understand why this is the case, moreover, I hope to illumine how our moral and religious presuppositions shape our medical care. Too often medicine becomes the means by which, in the name of humanity, we eliminate those who suffer. Thus, it has become common in our society to assume that certain children born with severe birth defects who also happen to be retarded should not be kept alive in order to spare them a lifetime of suffering. But why do we assume that it is the role of medicine to save us from suffering? By exploring whether we ought to try to eliminate the retarded I hope, therefore, to make explicit a whole set of assumptions about suffering and medicine's role in its alleviation.

Setting the Issues

Before addressing these large issues, however, I think it wise to discern more exactly some of the problems raised by the film as well as some of the problems of the film. It is obvious that the film is in serious conflict with the convictions of many who belong to and support the Association for Retarded Citizens. The film gives the impression that there is nothing more disastrous, nothing more destructive, than for a child to be born retarded, but the sponsoring organization for the film maintains that the retarded are not significantly different from the so-called normal. Indeed, the Association for Retarded Citizens believes that with appropriate training most retarded people can become contributing members of a society even as complex as our own. Thus the negative impression of retardation that the film conveys is not one which those sponsoring the film believe or think warranted. And it could have the unintended effect of reinforcing our society's largely negative attitude toward the retarded.

Perhaps, equally troubling is the indiscriminate use of the notion of "retardation" in the film. Not only does the film fail to denote the wide variety of retardation–sometimes much less serious than others–but even more it fails to make clear that our attribution of retardation may be due as much to our prejudices as it is the assumed limits of the retarded. It has become increasingly recognized that disease descriptions and remedies are relative to a society's values and needs. Thus, "retardation" might not "exist" in a society which values cooperation more than competition and ambition.

Yet the increasing realization that retardation is a social designation should not blind us to the fact that the retarded do have some quite specifiable problems peculiar to them and that their difference requires special forms of care. It is extremely important how we put this if we are to avoid two different perils. The first, assuming that societal prejudice is embodied in all designations of retardation, seeks to aid the retarded by preventing discriminatory practices in a manner similar to the civil rights campaigns for blacks and women. Because the retarded are said to have the same rights as anyone, in this view all they require is to be treated "normally." Without denying that the retarded have "rights" or that much good has been done under the banner "normalization," I believe this way of putting the matter is misleading and risks making the retarded subject to even greater societal cruelty (Hoffmaster 1982). Would it not be unjust to treat the retarded "equally"? Instead, retardation ought to be so precisely understood that those who are thus handicapped can be accommodated as they need. But that may be a reason for avoiding the word *retardation* altogether. As I have already noted there are so many different ways of being retarded, so many different kinds of disabilities and corresponding forms of care required that to isolate a group as "retarded" may be the source of much of the injustice we perpetrate on those whom we identify as "not normal."

The second peril is that of oppressive care, a kind of care based on the assumption that the retarded are so disabled they must be protected from the dangers and risks of life. Such a strategy subjects the retarded to a cruelty fuelled by our sentimental concern to deal with their differences by treating them as something less than human agents. Too often this strategy isolates the retarded from the rest of society in the interest of "protecting" them from societal indifference. As a result they are trained to be retarded. The challenge is to know how to characterize retardation and to know what difference it should make, without our very characterizations being used as an excuse to treat the retarded unjustly. However, we see this is not just a problem for the retarded, but a basic problem of any society, since societies are only possible because we are all different in skills and different in needs (Hauerwas 1977). Societies must find ways to characterize and institutionalize those differences so that we see them as enhancing rather than diminishing each of our lives. From this perspective the retarded are a poignant test of a society's particular understanding of how our differences are relevant to and for achievement of a common good.

The various issues I have raised can be illustrated by pointing to one final fallacy that the film underwrites. It gives the impression that retardation is primarily a genetic problem recognized at, or soon after, birth. But that is simply not the case. Half the people who bear the label "retarded" do so as the result of some circumstance after their conception and/or birth. Many are retarded due to environmental, nutritional, and/or accidental causes. To suggest, therefore, that we can eliminate retardation by better prenatal care or more thorough genetic screening and counseling is a mistake. Even if we were all required to have genetic checks before being allowed to marry, we would still have some among us that we currently label as "retarded."

We must ask what the "prevent retardation" campaign would mean for this group? If a society were even partially successful in "eliminating" retardation, how would it regard those who have become retarded? Since retardation was eliminated on grounds of being an unacceptable way of being human, would the retarded who remain live in a society able to recognize the validity of their existence and willing to provide the care they require? Of course it might be suggested that with fewer retarded there would be more resources for the care of those remaining. That is no doubt true, but the question is whether there would be the moral will to direct those resources in their direction. Our present resources are more than enough to provide good care for the retarded. That we do not provide such care can be attributed to a lack of moral will and imagination. What will and imagination there is comes from those who have found themselves unexpectedly committed to care for a retarded person through birth or relation. Remove that and I seriously doubt whether our society will find the moral convictions necessary to sustain our alleged commitment to the retarded.

To reckon whether this is mere speculation, consider this thought experiment. We live at a time when it is possible through genetic screening to predict who has the greatest likelihood of having a retarded child, particularly if that person marries someone of similar genetic characteristics. It has become a general policy for most of the population to have such screening and to choose their marriage partner accordingly. Moreover, amniocentesis has become so routine that the early abortion of handicapped children has become the medical "therapy" of choice. How would such a society regard and treat a couple who refused to be genetically screened, who refused amniocentesis, and who might perhaps have a less than normal child? Would such a society be happy with the increased burden on its social and financial resources? Why should citizens support the birth and care of such a child when its existence could easily have been avoided? To care for such a child, to support such "irresponsible" parents, means only that the "truly" needy will be unjustly deprived of care in the interest of sustaining a child who will never "contribute to societal good." That such an attitude seems not unreasonable to many people also suggests that in our current situation a campaign to "prevent retardation" might have negative implications for those who are retarded, as well as those who may have the misfortune to be born retarded or become retarded in the future.

Suffering and the Retarded

But surely there is something wrong with these observations, as they seem to imply that since we can never ensure that no one will be born or become retarded, then we should not even try to prevent retardation. On such grounds it seems we cannot change our lives to ensure that few will be born retarded so that those who are retarded now and in the future will not be cruelly treated and may even receive better care. That is clearly a vicious and unworthy position. We rightly seek to prevent those forms of retardation that are preventable. To challenge that assumption would be equivalent to questioning our belief that the world is round or that love is a good thing. Like so many things that seem obvious, however, if we ask *why* they seem so, we are often unable to supply an answer. Perhaps they seem obvious precisely because they do not require a reason for holding them.

I suspect that at least part of the reason it seems so obvious that we ought to prevent retardation is the conviction that we ought to prevent suffering. No one should will that an animal should suffer gratuitously. No one should will that a child should endure an illness. No one should will that another person should suffer from hunger. No one should will that a child should be born retarded. That suffering should be avoided is a belief as deep as any we have. That someone born retarded suffers is obvious. Therefore if we believe we ought to prevent suffering, it seems we ought to prevent retardation. Yet like many other "obvious" beliefs, the assumption that suffering should *always* be prevented, if analysed, becomes increasingly less certain or at least involves unanticipated complexity. Just because it implies eliminating subjects who happen to be retarded should at least suggest to us that something is wrong with our straightforward assumption that suffering should always be avoided or, if possible, eliminated. This is similar to some justifications of suicide:

namely, in the interest of avoiding or ending suffering a subject wills no longer to exist. Just because in suicide there is allegedly a decision by the victim does not alter the comparison with some programs to prevent retardation: Both assume that certain forms of suffering are so dehumanizing that it is better not to exist.

As I have indicated above, this assumption draws upon some of our most profound moral convictions. Yet I hope to show that our assumption that suffering should *always* be prevented is a serious and misleading oversimplification. To show why this is the case a general analysis of suffering is required. We assume we know what suffering is because it is so common, but on analysis, suffering turns out to be an extremely elusive subject. Only once that analysis has been done will we be in a position to ask if the retarded suffer from being retarded or whether the problem is the suffering we feel the retarded cause us.

The Kinds and Ways of Suffering

"To suffer" means to undergo, to be subject. But we undergo much we do not call suffering. Suffering names those aspects of our lives that we undergo and which have a particularly negative sense. We suffer when what we undergo blocks our positive desires and wants. Suffering also carries a sense of "surdness": It denotes those frustrations for which we can give no satisfying explanation and which we cannot make serve some wider end. Suffering thus names a sense of brute power, that does violence to our best laid plans. It is not easily domesticated. Therefore, there can be no purely descriptive account of suffering, since every description necessarily entails some judgment about the value or purpose of certain states.

No doubt the intensity of our own suffering or of our sympathy for others' suffering has reinforced our assumptions that we have a firm grip on its meaning. Yet it is certainly not clear that the kind of suffering occasioned by starvation is the same as that of cancer, though each is equally terrifying in its relentless but slow resolution in death. It is interesting that we also use *suffer* in an active sense of "bearing with," permitting, or enduring. While such expressions do not eclipse the passive sense associated with suffering, they at least connote that we do not associate suffering only with that for which we can do nothing.

Perhaps, this is the clue we have been needing to understand better the nature of suffering. We must distinguish between those forms of suffering that happen to us and those that we bring on ourselves or that are requisite to our purposes and goals. Some suffering which befalls us is integral to our goals, only we did not previously realize it. We tend to associate pain, however, with that which happens to us, since it seems to involve that which stands as a threat to our goals and projects, rather than as some means to a further end. In like manner, we suffer from illness and accidents–thus our association of pain with sickness and physical trauma. Of course pain and illness are interrelated, because most of the time when we are ill we hurt, but it is also true that conceptually pain and illness seem to stand on that side of suffering that is more a matter of fate than choice.

This distinction helps us to see the wider meaning of suffering. We not only suffer from diseases, accidents, tornadoes, earthquakes, droughts, floods–all those things over which we have little control–but we also suffer from other people, from living here rather than there, from doing this kind of job–all matters we might avoid–because in these instances we see what we suffer as part of a large scheme. This latter sense of "suffer," moreover, seems more subjective, since what may appear as a problem for one may seem an opportunity for another. Not only is what we suffer relative to our projects, but how we suffer is relative to what we have or wish to be (Thomas 1979; Bernard 1981).

Without denying the importance of the distinction between forms of suffering that happen to us and those that we instigate as requisite to our goals, we would be mistaken to press it too hard. Once considered, it may not seem as evident or as helpful as it first appeared. For example, we often discuss how what at the time looked like something that happened to us–something we suffered–was in fact something we did, or at least chose not to avoid. Our increasing knowledge of the relation of illness to life-style is enough to make us think twice before drawing a hard and fast distinction between what happens to us and what we do.

But the situation is even more complex. We often find that essential in our response to suffering is the ability to make what happens to me mine. Cancer patients frequently testify to some sense of relief when they find out they have cancer. The very ability to name what they have seems to give them a sense of control or possession that replaces the undifferentiated fear they had been feeling. Pain and suffering alienate us from ourselves. They make us what we do not know. The task is to find the means to make that which is happening to me mine–to interpret its presence (even if such an interpretation is negative) as something I can claim as integral to my identity. No doubt our power to transform events into decisions can be the source of great self-deception, but it is also the source of our moral identity.

Please note: I am not suggesting that every form of pain or suffering can or should be seen as some good or challenge. Extreme suffering can as easily destroy as enhance. Nor do I suggest that we should be the kind of people who can transform any suffering into benefit. We rightly feel that some forms of suffering can only be acknowledged, not transformed. Indeed, at this point I am not making any normative recommendations about how we should respond to suffering, rather I am suggesting the distinction between the suffering which happens to us and the suffering which we accept as part of our projects is not as clear as it may at first seem. More important is the question of what kind of people we ought to be so that certain forms of suffering are not denied but accepted as part and parcel of our existence as moral agents.

In spite of our inability to provide a single meaning to the notion of suffering or to distinguish clearly between different kinds of suffering, I think this analysis has not been without important implications. It may well be that those forms of suffering we believe we should try to prevent or to eliminate are those that we think impossible to integrate into our projects, socially or individually. It is exactly those forms of suffering which seem to intrude uncontrollably into our lives which appear to be the most urgent candidates for prevention. Thus, our sense that we should try to prevent suffering turns out to mean that we should try to prevent those kinds of suffering that we do not feel can serve any human good.

Even this way of putting the matter may be misleading. Some may object that while it is certainly descriptively true that we find it hard to integrate certain kinds of suffering into our individual and social lives, that ought not be the case. The issue is not what we do, but rather who we ought to be in order to be capable of accepting all suffering as a necessary aspect of human existence. In viewing our life narrowly as a matter of purposes and accomplishments, we may miss our actual need for suffering, even apparently purposeless or counter-purposeful suffering. The issue is not whether retarded children can serve a human good, but whether we should be the kind of people, the kind of parents and communities that can receive, even welcome, them into our midst in a manner that allows them to flourish.

But it may be objected that although this latter way of putting the issue seems to embody the highest moral ideals, in fact, it is deeply immoral because the suggestion that all forms of suffering are capable of being given human meaning is destructive to the human project. Certain kinds of suffering–Hiroshima, Auschwitz, wars–are so horrible we are able to preserve our humanity only by denying them human significance. No "meaning" can be derived from the Holocaust except that we must do everything we can to see that it does not happen again. Perhaps individuals can respond to natural disasters such as hurricanes and floods in a positive manner, but humanly we are right to view these other destructions as a scourge which we will neither accept nor try to explain in some positive sense.

Our refusal to accept certain kinds of suffering, or to try to interpret them as serving some human purpose, is essential for our moral health. Otherwise, we would far too easily accept the causes of suffering rather than trying to eliminate or avoid them. Our primary business is not to accept suffering, but to escape it, both for our own sake and our neighbor's. Still, in the very attempt to escape suffering, do we not lose something of our own humanity? We rightly try to avoid unnecessary suffering, but it also seems that we are never quite what we should be until we recognize the necessity and inevitability of suffering in our lives.

To be human is to suffer. That sounds wise. That sounds right, that is, true to the facts. But we should not be too quick to affirm it as a norm. Questions remain as to what kind of suffering should be accepted and how it should be integrated into our lives. Moreover, prior to these questions is the even more challenging question of why suffering seems to be our fate. Even if I knew how to answer such questions, I could not try to address them in this paper. (Indeed, I suspect that there can be no general answer that does not mislead as much as it informs.) But perhaps by directing our attention toward the retarded we can better understand why and how suffering is never to be merely "accepted" and yet why it is unavoidable in our lives. In preparation for that discussion, I need to try to suggest why it is that suffering seems so unavoidable.

On Why We Suffer

To ask why we suffer makes the questioner appear either terribly foolish or extremely arrogant. It seems foolish to ask, since in fact we *do* suffer and no sufficient reason can be given to explain that fact. Indeed, if it were explained, suffering would be denied some of its power. The question seems arrogant because it seeks to put us in the position of eating from the tree of good and evil. Only God knows the answer to such questions.

Without denying that the question of why we suffer can be foolish and pretentious, I think it is worth asking since it has one obvious answer: We suffer because we are incomplete beings who depend on one another for our existence. Indeed, the matter can be put more strongly, since we depend upon others not only for our survival but also for our identity. Suffering is built into our condition because it is literally true that we exist only to the extent that we sustain, or "suffer" the existence of others and the others include not just others like us, but mountains, trees, animals, and so on.

This is exactly contrary to cherished assumptions. We believe that identity derives from our independence, our self-possession. As Arthur McGill suggests, we think "a person is real so far as he can draw a line around certain items—his body, his thoughts, his house—and claim them as his own" (McGill 1983, p. 89). Thus death becomes our ultimate enemy—the intimation involved in every form of suffering—because it is the ultimate threat to our identity. Again, as McGill suggests, that is why what we suffer so often seems to take proportions: Our neediness seems to make us helpless to what we undergo. In this sense, our "neediness" represents a fundamental *flaw* in our identity, a basic inability to rest securely with those things which are one's own and which lie inside the line between oneself and the rest of reality. Need forces the self to become open to the not-self; it requires every man to come to terms with the threats of demonic power (McGill 1983, p. 90).

The irony is, however, that our neediness is also the source of our greatest strength, for our need requires the cooperation and love of others from which derives our ability not only to live but to flourish. Our identity, far from deriving from our self-possession, or our self-control, comes from being "de-possessed" of those powers whose promise is only illusory. Believing otherwise, fearful of our sense of need, when we attempt to deny our reliance on others, we become all the more subject to those powers. As we shall see, this has particularly significant implications for our relations with the retarded, since we "naturally" disdain those who do not or cannot cover up their neediness. Prophet-like, the retarded only remind us of the insecurity hidden in our false sense of self-possession (Raine 1982).

It may be objected that such an account of suffering is falsely subtle, since it is obvious why we suffer: Bad things happen to us. We are injured in accidents; we lose everything in a flood; our community is destroyed by a tornado; we get cancer; a retarded child is born. These are not things that happen to us because of our needs, but rather they happen because they happen. Yet each does relate to concrete needs–the need for security and safety, the need for every-dayness, the need for health, the need for new life. If we try to deny any of these needs, as well as many others, we deny ourselves the necessary resources for well-lived lives and make ourselves all the more subject to the powers who draw their strength from our fears. I have not tried in this brief and inadequate account of why we suffer to offer anything like a theodicy. Indeed, I remain skeptical of all attempts to provide some general account or explanation of evil or suffering. For example, it is by no means clear that evil and suffering raise the same questions, since certainly not every form of suffering is evil. Moreover, as I have suggested above, I do not think any explanation that removes the surdness of certain forms of suffering can be right. Much in our lives should not be made "good" or explained. All I have tried to do is to state the obvious–we suffer because we are inherently creatures of need. This does not explain, much less justify our suffering or the evil we endure. But it does help us understand why the general policy to prevent suffering is at least odd as a general policy. Our task is to prevent unnecessary suffering, but the hard question, as we have seen, is to know what constitutes unnecessary suffering. It is even more difficult when the question concerns another, as it does in the case of the retarded. It is just that question to which we now must turn.

Do the Retarded Suffer from Being Retarded?

I suggested above that behind the claim that we ought to prevent retardation lies the assumption that we ought to prevent suffering or, in particular, unnecessary suffering. I have tried at least to raise some critical questions about that assumption. But there is another issue that requires equal analysis. Are we right to assume that the retarded are suffering by being, retarded? Certainly they suffer retardation, but do they suffer from being retarded?

No doubt, like everyone, the retarded suffer. Like us, they have accidents. Like us, they have colds, sores, and cancer. Like us, they are subject to natural disasters. Like us, they die. But the question is whether they suffer from being retarded. We assume they suffer because of their retardation, just as we or others suffer from being born blind or deaf. Yet it is by no means clear that such cases are similar or even whether those born blind or deaf suffer from blindness or deafness. It is possible that they are in fact taught by us that they are decisively disabled, and thus learn to suffer. If that is the case, then there is at least some difference between going blind and being retarded, since the very nature of being retarded means there is a limit to their understanding of their disadvantage and thus the extent of their suffering. That may also be true of being blind or deaf, of course, but not in the same way.

Do the retarded understand that they are retarded? Certainly most are able to see that they are different than many of us, but there is no reason to think they would on their own come to understand their condition as "retardation" or that they are in some decisive way suffering. They may perceive that there are some things some people do easily which they can do only with great effort or not at all, but that in itself is not sufficient reason to attribute to them great suffering. Of course it may be objected that if we are to care for them, if we are to help alleviate some of the results of their being retarded, we cannot help but try to make them understand their limits. We have to make them conscious of their retardation if we are to help them be free from some of the effects of their condition. But again, this is certainly not as clear as it first appears, for it by no means follows that by learning to confront their limits in order to better their life, the retarded necessarily understand they are thereby suffering from something called "retardation," "Down's Syndrome," or the like.

Yet we persist in the notion that the retarded are suffering and suffering so much from being retarded that it would be better for them not to exist than to have to bear such disability. It is important I not be misunderstood. I am not suggesting that retardation is a minor problem or that nothing should be done to try to prevent, alleviate, or lessen the effects of being retarded; I have tried, rather, to suggest that the widespread assumption that the retarded suffer from being retarded is by no means obviously true.

Perhaps, what we assume is not that the retarded suffer from being retarded but rather, because they are retarded they will suffer from being in a world like ours. They will suffer from inadequate housing, inadequate medical care, inadequate schooling, lack of love and care. They will suffer from discrimination as well as cruel kidding and treatment from unfeeling peers. All this is certainly true, but it is not an argument for preventing retardation in the name of preventing suffering; rather it is an argument for changing the nature of the world in the interest of preventing the needless suffering we impose on the retarded.

It may be observed that we have very little hope that the world will or can be changed in this respect, but even if that is the case it would be insufficient grounds for the general policy of eliminating the retarded. On such grounds anyone suffering injustice or ill-treatment would be in jeopardy. If justice comes to mean the elimination of the victim of injustice rather than the cause of injustice, we stand the risk of creating admittedly a less troubled but deeply unjust world.

The need to subject this set of assumptions to rigorous analysis is particularly pressing in relation to the care of children born retarded or otherwise handicapped. A policy of non-treatment is often justified as a means of sparing a child a life of suffering. I by no means wish to argue that every child should receive the most energetic medical care to keep it alive, but if such care is withheld it cannot be simply to spare the child a life of suffering. On such grounds few children with any moderately serious chronic health problem would be cared for at birth. We all, healthy and non-healthy, normal or abnormal, are destined for a life of suffering.

Some will say that this is surely to miss the point behind the concern to spare certain children a life of suffering. The issue is the extent and intensity of the suffering. But again, such a judgment is a projection of our assumptions about how we would feel if we were in their situation. But that is exactly what we are not. We do not know to what extent they may suffer from their disability. We do not know how much pain they will undergo, but we nonetheless act to justify our lack of care in the name of our humane concern about their destiny. We do so even knowing that our greatest nobility as humans often derives from the individual's struggle to make positive use of his or her limitations.

I am not suggesting, that the care we give to severely disabled children (or adults) will always result in happy results for themselves or those around them. But to refrain from such care to spare them future suffering can be a formula for profound self-deception. Too often the suffering we wish to spare them is the result of our unwillingness to change our lives so that those disabled might have a better life. Or, even more troubling, we refrain from life-giving care simply because we do not like to have those who are different from us to care for.

Our Suffering of the Retarded

Why, therefore, do we persist in assumptions that the retarded suffer from being retarded? At least something of an answer comes from a most unlikely source: Adam Smith's *Theory of Moral Sentiments*. In that book Smith endeavours to provide an account for why, no matter how "selfish a man may be supposed, there are evidently some principles in his nature which interest him in the fortune of others, and render their happiness necessary to him, though he derives nothing from it except the pleasure of seeing it" (Smith 1976, p. 1, 11). Such a sentiment, Smith observes, is by no means confined to the virtuous, since even the most "hardened ruffian" at times may derive sorrow from the sorrow of others. Still, according to Smith, this is something of a puzzle. Since we have no "immediate experience of what other men feel, we can form no idea of the manner in which they are affected, but by conceiving what we ourselves should feel in the like situation. Though our brother is upon the rack, as long as we ourselves are at our case, our senses will never inform us what he suffers. They never did, and never can, carry us beyond our own person, and it is by the imagination only that we can form any conception of what are his sensations" (Smith 1976, p. 1, 2).

It is through our imagination, therefore, that our fellow-feeling with the sorrow of others is generated. But our sympathy does not extend to every passion, for there are some passions that disgust us–thus, the furious behavior of an angry man may actually make us more sympathetic with his enemies. That this is so makes us especially anxious to be people capable of eliciting sympathy from others, thus "sympathy enlivens joy and alleviates grief. It enlivens joy by presenting another source of satisfaction; and it alleviates grief by insinuating unto the heart almost the only agreeable sensation which it is at that time capable of receiving" (Smith 1976, p. 1, 1). By knowing our sorrow is shared by another we seem to be less burdened with our distress. Moreover, we are pleased when we are able to sympathize with one who is suffering, but we look forward more to enjoying another's good fortune.

Because we seek to sympathize as well as be the object of sympathy, Smith observes:

Of all the calamities to which the condition of mortality exposes mankind, the loss of reason appears, to those who have the least spark of humanity, by far the most dreadful, and they behold that last stage of human "wretchedness" with deeper commiseration than any other. But the poor wretch, who is in it, laughs and sings perhaps, and is altogether insensible of his own misery. The anguish which humanity feels, therefore, at the sight of such an object, cannot be the reflection of any sentiment of the sufferer. The compassion of the spectator must arise altogether from the consideration of what he himself would feel if he was reduced to the same unhappy situation, and, what perhaps is impossible, was at the same time able to regard it with his present reason and judgment. (Smith 1976, p. 1, 11)

We thus persist in our assumption that the retarded suffer from being retarded not because we are unsympathetic with them but because we are not sure how to be sympathetic with them. We fear that the very imagination which is the source of our sympathy, on which our fellow feeling is founded, is not shared by them. To lack such an important resource, we suspect, means they are fatally flawed, for one thus lacks the ability to be the subject of sympathy. We seek to prevent retardation not because we are inhumane but because we feel the retarded lack the means of giving and receiving sympathy, and thus we cannot imagine how they feel. Exactly because we are unsure they have the capacity to suffer as we suffer, we seek to avoid their presence in order to avoid the limits of our own sympathy.

As Smith observes, we have no way to know what the retarded suffer as retarded. All we know is how we imagine we would feel if we were retarded. We thus often think we would rather not exist at all than to exist as one retarded. As a result, we miss the point at issue. For the retarded do not feel or understand their retardation as we do, or imagine we would, but rather as they do. We have no right or basis to attribute our assumed unhappiness or suffering to them. Ironically, therefore, the policy of preventing suffering is one based on a failure of imagination. Unable to see like the retarded, to hear like the retarded, we attribute to them our suffering. We thus rob them of the opportunity to do what each of us must do–learn to bear and live with our individual sufferings.

Need, Loneliness, and the Retarded

In many respects, however, our inability to sympathize with the retarded–to see their life as they see it, to suffer their suffering–is but an aspect of a more general problem. As Smith observes, we do not readily expose our sufferings, because none of us are anxious to identify with the sufferings of others. We try to present a pleasant appearance in order to elicit fellow-feeling with others. We fear to be sufferers, to be in pain, to be unpleasant, because we fear so desperately the loss of fellow-feeling on the part of others. We resent those who suffer without apology, as we expect the sufferer at least to show shame in exchange for our sympathy.

As much as we fear suffering, we fear more the loneliness that accompanies it. We try to deny our neediness as much, if not more so, to ourselves as to others. We seek to be strong. We seek to be self-possessed. We seek to deny that we depend on others for our existence. We will be self-reliant and we resent and avoid those who do not seek to be like us–the strong. We will be friends to one another only so long as we promise not to impose seriously our sufferings on the others. Of course, we willingly enter into some of our friends' suffering–indeed to do so only reinforces our sense of strength-but we expect such suffering to be bounded by a more determinative strength.

That we avoid the sufferer is not because we are deeply unsympathetic or inhumane, but because of the very character of suffering. By its very nature suffering alienates us not only from one another but from ourselves, especially suffering which we undergo, which is not easily integrated into our ongoing projects or hopes. To suffer is to have our identity threatened physically, psychologically, and morally. Thus our suffering even makes us unsure of who we are.

It is not surprising, therefore, that we should have trouble with the suffering of others. None of us willingly seeks to enter into the loneliness of others. We fear such loneliness may result in loss of control of our own life. We feel we must be very strong to be able to help the weak and needy. We may be right about that, but we may also fail to understand the kind of help they really need. Too often we seek to do something rather than first simply learn how to be with, to be present to, the sufferer in his or her loneliness. We especially fear, if not dislike, those whose suffering is the kind for which we can do nothing.

The retarded, therefore, are particularly troubling for us. Even if they do not suffer by being retarded, they are certainly people in need. Even worse, they do not try to hide their needs. They are not self-sufficient, they are not self-possessed, they are in need. Even more, they do not evidence the proper shame for being so. They simply assume that they are what they are and they need to provide no justification for being such. It is almost as if they have been given a natural grace to be free from the regret most of us feel for our neediness.

That such is the case, however, does not mean that the retarded do not suffer from the general tendency of wanting to be self-sufficient. Like us they are more than capable of engaging in the self-deceptive project of being their own person. Nor is such an attempt entirely wrong, for they, like us, rightly seek to develop skills that can help them help themselves as well as others. Yet we perceive them as essentially different from us, as beings whose condition has doomed them to a loneliness we fear worse than suffering itself, and, as a result, we seek to prevent retardation.

That we are led to such an extreme derives partly from our frustration at not being able to cure the retarded. We seek to help them overcome their disability, but we know that even our best efforts will not result in the retarded not being retarded. After all, what we finally seek is not simply to help the retarded better negotiate their disability but to be like us: not retarded. Our inability to accomplish that frustrates and angers us, and sometimes the retarded themselves become the object of our anger. We do not like to be reminded of the limits of our power, and we do not like those who remind us.

We fervently seek to help the retarded, to *do for* the retarded, to make their lot less subject to suffering. No doubt much good derives from such efforts. But our frenzied activity can also be a failure to recognize that our attempts to help, our attempt "to do for" the retarded must first be governed by our ability to be "with" the retarded. Only as we learn to be and do with the retarded, do we learn that their retardation, our projection of their suffering, need not create an unbridgeable gap between them and us. We learn that they are not incapable of fellow-feeling with us and, just as important, that we are not incapable of fellow-feeling with them.

That such fellow-feeling is possible does not mean that they are "really just like us." They are not. They do not have the same joys we have nor do they suffer just as we suffer. But in our joys and in our sufferings they recognize something of their joy and their suffering, and they offer to share their neediness with us. Such an offer enables us in quite surprising ways to discover that we have needs to share with them. We are thus freed from the false and vicious circle of having to appear strong before others' weakness, and we are then able to join with the retarded in the common project of sharing our needs and satisfactions. As a result we discover we no longer fear them.

I am not suggesting that such sharing comes easily. Few of us are prepared to enter naturally into such a life. Indeed most of us, cherishing the illusion of our strength, must be drawn in reluctantly. But miraculously many are so graced. Day in and day out, through life with their retarded child, brother, or friend, they learn to see themselves through the eyes of the other who happens also to be retarded. Moreover, by learning not to fear the other's retardation, they learn not to fear their own neediness.

Thus if we are to make a movie to help others avoid unnecessary risks that can result in retardation, let us not begin soon after the birth. To begin there is grossly unfair, because it catches us before we are even sure what has happened to us. Let the film begin several years after the birth, after the parents of a child born retarded have discovered, like all parents must, that they are capable of dealing with this. It is not the child they would have willed, but then all children turn out to be different than our expectations. This child, to be sure, raises particular challenges, but let the film show the confidence of the couple that comes from facing those challenges. Unless suggestions for avoiding retarded children are bounded by such confidence, we cannot help but make the life of the retarded that much more difficult. But even more destructive, such a campaign is bound to make our own illusory fears of the retarded and our own needs that much more powerful.

An Inconclusive Theological Postscript

It may well be asked what all this has to do with our religious convictions as Christians. Of course, some obvious connections can be drawn. Christians are alleged to be concerned with the weak and the downtrodden. The retarded seem to fit that description. Since the position developed generally supports the ideal of help for the retarded, it seems consistent with such a religious sentiment. Or it may be suggested that Christians are a people who have learned to accept that life is under God's direction. They attribute to God the bad as well as the good. Parents, in particular, think it presumptuous to try to determine the quality of their offspring. They accept their retarded, as well as their more nearly normal children, as God's will. They do not presume arrogantly to ask why, or to what purpose, retarded children are born.

There is some truth to each of these positions, but they have to be stated much more carefully. Concern with the downtrodden can too easily result in sentimental acceptance and care of the retarded that fails to respect the integrity of their existence. It condemns the retarded to being "weak" so that they might receive our "charity" rather than acknowledging them to be essential members of our community. The second position, God's will, has been and is used wrongly to justify acceptance of avoidable suffering and injustice.

Yet these more obvious theological connections are not the most significant for helping us understand how we as Christians should respond to the retarded. Quite simply, the challenge of learning to know, to be with, and care for the retarded is nothing less than learning to know, be with, and love God. God's face is the face of the retarded; God's body is the body of the retarded; God's being is that of the retarded. For the God we Christians must learn to worship is not a god of self-sufficient power, a god who in self-possession needs no one; rather ours is a God who needs a people, who needs a son. Absoluteness of being or power is not a work of the God we have come to know through the cross of Christ (McGill 1983, p. 75).

Arthur McGill has perceptively interpreted the classical trinitarian debate in this fashion. He suggests:

The issue between Arius and Athansius has nothing to do with whether God is one or two or three. It has to do with what quality makes God divine, what quality constitutes his perfection. From the perspective of self-contained absoluteness and transcendent supremacy, Arius can only look upon God's begetting a Son as grotesque blasphemy. God, he observed, must be very imperfect if he must generate a Son in order to become complete. But from the perspective of self-communicating love, Athanasius can look upon the dependent derived Son, not as a blot upon God's divinity, but as a mode of its perfection. Love and not transcendence, giving and not being superior, are qualities that mark God's divinity. Since giving entails receiving, there must be a receptive, dependent, needy pole within the being of God. It is pride–and not love–that fears dependence and that worships transcendence. (McGill 1983, p. 78)

That is why in the face of the retarded we are offered an opportunity to see God, for like God they offer us an opportunity of recognizing the character of our neediness. In truth the retarded in this respect are but an instance of the capacity we each have for one another. That the retarded are singled out is only an indication of how they can serve for us all as a prophetic sign of our true nature as creatures destined to need God and, thus, one another.

Moreover, it is through such a recognition that we learn how God would have the world governed. As we are told in the Epistle to Diognetus in answer to the question of why God sent his Son: "to rule as a tyrant, to inspire terror and astonishment? No, he did not. No, he sent him in gentleness and mildness. To be sure, as a king sending his royal son, he sent him as God. But he sent him as to men, as saving and persuading them, and not as exercising force. For force is no attribute to God" (McGill 1983, p. 82). But if force is no attribute of God's governance, suffering is. Unlike us, God is not separated from himself or us by his suffering; rather, his suffering makes it possible for him to share our life and for us to share his.

Learning to share our life with God is no doubt difficult–it must be at least as demanding as learning that we can share life with the retarded. But that such a sharing of our sufferings as well as our joys is necessary cannot be doubted. For a world where there is no unpatterned, unpurposeful suffering would be devoid of the means for us to grow out of our selfishness and into love. That is why those who worship such a God are obligated to be confident that we can live well with those whose difference from ourselves we have learned to characterize by the unfortunate label, "retarded." For if we did not so learn to live, we know we would be decisively retarded: retarded in our ability to turn ourselves to other's needs, regardless of the cost.

REFERENCES

Hauerwas, Stanley (1977). 'Community and Diversity: The Tyranny of Normality.' *National Apostolate for the Mentally Retarded*, 8 1-2, pp. 20-22.

Hauerwas, Stanley (1979). 'Reflections on Suffering, Death, and Medicine.' *Ethics in Science and Medicine*, 6, pp. 229-237.

Hoffmaster, Barry (1982). 'Caring for Retarded Persons: Ideals and Practical Choices.' In Stanley Hauerwas (Ed). *Responsibility for Devalued Persons: Ethical Interactions Between Society, the Family, and the Retarded*, pp. 24-38. Springfield, Illinois: Charles Thomas Press.

McGill, Arthur (1983). *Suffering, A Test Case of Theological Method*. Philadelphia: Westminster Press.

Nagel, Thomas (1979). *Mortal Questions*. Cambridge: Cambridge University Press. See especially pp. 24-38.

Raine, Bonita (1982). 'Care and Mentally Retarded People: Pastoral Dimensions Appropriate to Christian Ethical Convictions.' Dissertation, University of Notre Dame.

Smith, Adam (1976). *The Theory of Moral Sentiments*. D. D. Raphael and A. L. Macfie (Eds.). Oxford: Oxford University Press.

Williams, Bernard (1981). *Moral Luck*. Cambridge: Cambridge University Press.

Response:
Thoughts on Suffering:
A Parent's View

Hazel Morgan

SUMMARY. This paper concurs with Professor Hauerwas' strong misgivings about policies to prevent learning disabilities per se. It explores the link between suffering and having a learning disability, agreeing with the view that suffering is often caused by attitudes within society. It emphasises that there needs to be empathy with the aspirations of people with learning disabilities; that paternalist attitudes are unacceptable and that there needs to be reciprocity in relationships. It argues strongly against viewing people with learning disabilities as a homogeneous group. *[Article copies available for a fee from The Haworth Document Delivery Service: 1-800-HAWORTH. E-mail address: <docdelivery@haworthpress.com> Website: <http://www.HaworthPress.com> © 2004 by The Haworth Press, Inc. All rights reserved.]*

KEYWORDS. Learning disability, suffering, community, parenting

---

Hazel Morgan is the Head of the Foundation for People with Learning Disabilities in London. She has extensive experience of working with people with learning disabilities in a professional capacity and as a parent of a son with severe and complex needs.

[Haworth co-indexing entry note]: "Response: Thoughts on Suffering: A Parent's View." Morgan, Hazel. Co-published simultaneously in *Journal of Religion, Disability & Health* (The Haworth Pastoral Press, an imprint of The Haworth Press, Inc.) Vol. 8, No. 3/4, 2004, pp. 107-112; and: *Critical Reflections on Stanley Hauerwas' Theology of Disability: Disabling Society, Enabling Theology* (ed: John Swinton) The Haworth Pastoral Press, an imprint of The Haworth Press, Inc., 2004, pp. 107-112. Single or multiple copies of this article are available for a fee from The Haworth Document Delivery Service [1-800-HAWORTH, 9:00 a.m. - 5:00 p.m. (EST). E-mail address: docdelivery@haworthpress.com].

Digital Object Identifier: 10.1300/J095v8n03_12

I approach Professor Hauerwas' work from the perspective of a mother whose younger son, Peter, had Down's syndrome and additional disabilities. He sadly died in 1995 at the age of eighteen, having suffered massive strokes 11 months previously. I also bring a professional perspective as Head of the Foundation for People with Learning Disabilities, part of the Mental Health Foundation, a UK charity which funds research and community development projects, disseminates their findings and seeks to influence policy. Throughout this response I shall be using the term learning disability, as for many, retardation is not now an acceptable term.

I wish to explore four issues from the chapter, Suffering the Retarded: Should we prevent retardation?

- Concern about preventing learning disability, the message of the film described in the first paragraphs.
- The link between learning disability and suffering.
- The attitudes of other people towards disability.
- Whether it is desirable, as the chapter does, to generalise about people with learning disabilities and their parents.

I share Professor Hauerwas' concern at the implications of the film he narrates and his view that something is wrong with a general policy that seeks to prevent learning disability per se. Everyone would advocate good and responsible prenatal care and improved social conditions to reduce the incidence of disability. However, I have profound concern about the policies which have intensified in many areas since 1986 to eliminate disability through prenatal screening. Although offered in the name of "choice," there are many pressures on parents to accept the termination of pregnancies, not least because the birth of a disabled baby is so frequently regarded as a tragedy. This was illustrated recently by a legal case in which a mother gained undisclosed damages after physicians delayed an emergency caesarean operation without consulting her on the grounds that they assumed she would not want a severely disabled son. The woman claimed that her autonomy had been infringed and that she would have preferred to have had the baby 'regardless of any condition he was in.' Her baby was then still born (www.buryfreepress.co.uk 20/02/02). Professor Hauerwas' reminder that we should be uneasy about blanket statements on the desirability of eliminating disability is even more pertinent today than it might have been when the essay was originally written.

Hauerwas argues that the motivation for prevention is often partly to eliminate suffering. He contends, "that someone born retarded suffers is obvious." He distinguishes between suffering that happens to us from what might be termed as fate, cancer, or floods from suffering that derives from circumstances in which we live, which can sometimes be changed. When people have learning disabilities, there is often physical suffering; for example, people with Down's syndrome are more likely to have heart problems or hearing loss. I cannot deny that Peter had an unusually hard and difficult time and in the last months of his life was paralysed, and had a trachaeostomy and gastrostomy. Yet once his condition had stabilised after his strokes and he could be moved to the Sue Ryder Home he gave every indication that he enjoyed the music he listened to, the companionship of the staff and the visits of family and friends. As the consultant psychiatrist who visited him said, from a long career she had many memories of people with Down's syndrome, but she would never forget his hold on life against all the odds.

Much suffering for people with learning disabilities derives from people's attitudes, not least in relation to the whole question of eliminating disability. The Foundation has been conducting an enquiry into meeting the mental health needs of young people with learning disabilities. Some of the evidence being presented to the expert committee was about the pain being experienced by young people with learning disabilities in knowing that there are those who think they should have not been born. The evidence would also suggest that some young people *do* suffer from a perception that they are different and have different opportunities, particularly if they have mild learning disabilities. As we thankfully move towards a more inclusive society, how inclusion occurs is crucial. I believe that people with severe learning disabilities are also aware of the attitudes of others. I take Peter as an example. As he did not talk I do not know how far he was aware of difference, but I imagine he was hurt when parents moved their children away from him as he paddled at the edge of the sea. Again he was likely to have been upset when a Vicar asked us to take him out of a service at which a famous Christian orchestra had been invited to play. We need greater sensitivity and awareness in society.

Professor Hauerwas may be correct when he questions the widespread assumption that those with learning disabilities suffer from having this disability in itself. It is hard nonetheless to untangle the factors that impinge on people's lives whether from physical suffering or the attitudes of others, but none of these can lend support to an argument that suggest that these lives are not worth living. In considering the extent of the suffering of people with learning disabilities Professor Hauerwas makes a powerful case for improving society to lessen hardship and promote justice. That is what those of us who are involved in voluntary organisations are seeking to do, whether by campaigning, demonstrating innovative service models, promoting good practice or more respectful policies. He writes, "Too often the suffering we wish to spare them is the result of our unwillingness to change our lives so that those disabled might have a better life." This is a vital point, the implications of which should not be overlooked.

However, in considering attitudes towards those who have a learning disability, I would certainly take issue with the statement by Professor Hauerwas that "bad things happen to us, we are injured in accidents, a retarded child is born." I know that when I look back in old age that I will count the eighteen years spent with Peter among the richest of my life, as we shared his enjoyment of celebrations, outings, picnics, friendships and, above all, music. Peter's life was *not* a bad thing on par with accidents and illness. Quite the opposite, we shared love, sadness and happiness; he taught us so much.

Professor Hauerwas highlights an interesting tension in our western societies. Since the eighteenth century Enlightenment there has been an increasing emphasis on individuality and autonomy. This is challenged by disability in which there is likely to be a level of dependence. Old age is feared for similar reasons. He suggests, however, that it is in relationship to one another that we define our identity and that our neediness for the love and cooperation of others enables us not only to live but also to flourish. Yet we prefer to appear self-sufficient. People with learning disabilities do not usually have this option.

He discusses how sympathy enables us to share in one another's suffering, but our perception is coloured by our own personal views. Therefore, we imagine what we would feel ourselves if we had learning disabilities and because this is so hard it makes us feel uncomfortable. This can lead to a justification for seeking to eliminate the disabled baby. In the Preface to *Through Peter's Eyes*, Professor Hauerwas writes, "we confront the attitude that it would be better if such children did not exist–the attitude that often appears as compassion but actually denies their existence. Mrs. Morgan . . . will not let us still Peter's voice . . . " (Morgan 1990, p. vii).

In my experience discussions about disability often focus on the issue of quality of life and this was exemplified in the case of Dr. Arthur in 1981. He was put on trial for manslaughter 'for allowing baby John Pearson to die' when his parents rejected him on account of his Down's syndrome (Morgan 1990, p. 16). In the media coverage that followed there was a great deal of discussion of quality of life. We as a society bear much of the responsibility for the life experiences of disabled people; we also have no right to make these judgements about the internal experiences of others. For someone with severe learning disabilities, does not love, friendship, music, celebrations, the enjoyment of the bustle of the town, or the peace of the countryside constitute the foundations for a good life? It was our impression that these were important to Peter and my friendship with other people with learning disabilities has done nothing to lessen this conviction.

In the last section of the chapter, Professor Hauerwas discusses need, lone-liness, and 'the retarded.' Rightly, in my view, he suggests that the way for-ward is not to do good in a paternalist fashion, but to learn how to be with. Much of our life with Peter was being with him, sitting alongside him as he lis-tened to his favourite music, the Rachmaninov or the Vivaldi tapes, sharing his pleasure of a ride in the car along the country lanes of East Anglia. Following his strokes during the months in hospital and in the Sue Ryder Home, most of his physical care was no longer in our hands, but in the hands of health profes-sionals. We had to accustom ourselves just to being with him and offering our love. We all needed to be together as much as possible. I recognised my own neediness for companionship with Peter. Since Peter's death my life has been lived at a much faster pace and I am losing this capacity just to be with which I learnt and valued for eighteen years. There is an enormous challenge in the post industrial age to have time to be with one another.

The aspects of the essay with which I am least comfortable are those which stereotype people with learning disabilities and their families. In the notes to the chapter, Professor Hauerwas implies that all parents are frustrated by the presence of a retarded child. He suggests that the frustration derives from the fact that they cannot get better, although they learn that progress can be made and come to appreciate this. I am not sure this is always the case. Parents vary and many love and accept their son or daughter from the moment they are born and frustration is not the appropriate word in all cases.

With respect to people with learning disabilities, I would question Profes-sor Hauerwas' assertion that "they do not have the same joys we have nor do they suffer just as we suffer." How can such a sweeping judgement be made? Each of us, whoever we are, experience life uniquely. The research that we have carried out at the Foundation for People with Learning Disabilities in re-cent years has indicated that people with learning disabilities seek the life ex-periences of life as others in their community. "People with severe disabilities are buying their own homes, eating out, going to concerts, attending college, going to places of worship, getting to conferences" (Mental Health Founda-tion 1996, p. 103). Written ten years after the essay, this painted a picture of a life of greater opportunity, but it also recognised that many live in poverty, have little meaningful activity during the day, few friends.

Rather than seeing people with learning disabilities as a homogeneous group, I would argue that it is more helpful to see each person as having in-dividual gifts and needs. In *Everyday Lives, Everyday Choices* (FPLD 2000, p. 66) reported on projects exploring how people with learning dis-abilities who use few or no words could bring changes to their lives. Mandy Neville, Director of Circles Network, in an introduction to a chapter on friendship reflected on the appreciation of difference.

"In creating inclusive communities where people are welcomed for whom they are, where friendships are based on love and not on paid exchange and where differences are seen to be gifts we each will experience new ways to think and behave." When we received the diagnosis that our son had Down's syndrome this dominated our thoughts for a few days, but then he was Peter, and his disability was secondary. He brought us great joy and we trust that this was reciprocated. It seems to me that this is the secret: not to seek to label but to view each relationship as unique and infinitely valuable.

REFERENCES

Foundation for People with Learning Disabilities (2000). *Everyday Lives, Everyday Choices for People with Learning Disabilities, and High Support Needs*. London: The Mental Health Foundation.
Mental Health Foundation (1996). *Building Expectations: Opportunities and services for adults with a learning disability*. London: The Mental Health Foundation.
Morgan, H. (1990). *Through Peter's Eyes*. London: Arthur James.

Chapter 6

Must a Patient Be a Person
to Be a Patient?
Or, My Uncle Charlie
Is Not Much of a Person
But He Is Still
My Uncle Charlie

Stanley Hauerwas, PhD

[Originally published in *Connecticut Medicine* 39 December 1975, 39815, 17.] Reprinted with permission.

SUMMARY. Hauerwas urges us to move away from the concept of the 'person.' He suggests that the concept of 'person' is inadequate but probably also misleading and even dangerous. As a regulative notion to define the relation between doctor and patient the concept of person not only does violence to our language but fails to provide sufficient moral content to the practice of medicine and health care. He argues that the

---

[Haworth co-indexing entry note]: "Must a Patient Be a Person to Be a Patient? Or, My Uncle Charlie Is Not Much of a Person But He Is Still My Uncle Charlie." Hauerwas, Stanley. Co-published simultaneously in *Journal of Religion, Disability & Health* (The Haworth Pastoral Press, an imprint of The Haworth Press, Inc.) Vol. 8, No. 3/4, 2004, pp. 113-119; and: *Critical Reflections on Stanley Hauerwas' Theology of Disability: Disabling Society, Enabling Theology* (ed: John Swinton) The Haworth Pastoral Press, an imprint of The Haworth Press, Inc., 2004, pp. 113-119. Single or multiple copies of this article are available for a fee from The Haworth Document Delivery Service [1-800-HAWORTH, 9:00 a.m. - 5:00 p.m. (EST). E-mail address: docdelivery@haworthpress.com].

concept of 'person' not only suffers from abstraction by taking us out of the concrete social structure (community) and historical narrative (story) in which humans live, but can actually distort the practices, institutions and notions which underlay how we have learned morally to display our lives. While the idea of the 'person' can act as a moral restraint for some of the excesses of medical technology, its parameters often exclude, rather than include, people with disabilities. Hauerwas argues that in the absence of a shared moral vision for medical practices the concept of the person is questionable and perhaps even dangerous. He calls Christians and Jews to re-think the moral basis of medicine and to practice a form of medicine which is faithful to their traditions.

KEYWORDS. Person, personhood, medicine, disability

As a Protestant teaching at a Catholic university, I continue to learn about problems I had no idea even existed. For example, recently I was called down for referring to Catholics as "Roman Catholics." I had been working on the assumption that a Catholic was a Roman Catholic; however, it was pointed out to me that this phrase appeared only with the beginning of the English reformation in order to distinguish a Roman from an Anglo-Catholic. A Catholic is not Roman, as my Irish Catholic friend emphatically reminded me, but is more properly thought of simply as a Catholic.

I recount this tale because I think it has something to do with the issue I want to raise for our consideration. For we tend to think that most of our descriptions, the way we individuate action, have a long and honored history that can he tampered with only with great hesitation. Often, however, the supposed tradition is a recent innovation that may be as misleading as it is helpful.

That is what I think may be happening with the emphasis on whether someone is or is not a "person" when this is used to determine whether or what kind of medical care a patient should receive. In the literature of past medical ethics the notion of "person" does not seem to have played a prominent role in deciding how medicine should or should not be used vis-à-vis a particular patient. Why is it then that we suddenly seem so concerned with the question of whether someone is a person? It is my hunch we have much to learn from this phenomenon as it is an indication, not that our philosophy of medicine or medical ethics is in good shape, but rather that it is in deep trouble. For it is my thesis that we are trying to put forward "person" as a regulative notion to direct our health care as substitute for what only a substantive community and story can do.

However, before trying to defend this thesis, let me first illustrate how the notion of "person" is being used in relation to some of the recent issues of medical ethics. Paul Ramsey in his book, *The Patient as Person* (Ramsey 1970), uses the notion of person to protect the individual patient against the temptation, especially in experimental medicine, to use one patient for the good of another or society. According to Ramsey, the major issue of medical ethics is how to reconcile the welfare of the individual with the welfare of mankind when both must he served. Ramsey argues that it is necessary to emphasize the personhood of the patient in order to remind the doctor or the experimenter that his first responsibility is to his immediate patient, not mankind or even the patient's family. Thus, Ramsey's emphasis on "person" is an attempt to provide the basis for what he takes to be the central ethical commitment of medicine, namely, that no man will be used as a means for the good of another. Medicine can serve mankind only as it does so through serving the individual patient.

Without the presumption of the inviolability of the "person" Ramsey thinks that we would have no basis for "informed consent" as the controlling criteria for medical therapy and experimentation. Moreover, it is only on this basis that doctors rightly see that their task is not to cure diseases, but rather to cure the person who happens to be subject to a disease. Thus, the notion of "person" functions for Ramsey as a Kantian or deontological check on what he suspects is the utilitarian bias of modern medicine.

However, the notion of "person" plays quite a different function in other literature dealing with medical ethics. In these contexts, "person" is not used primarily as a protective notion, but rather as a permissive notion that takes the moral heat off certain quandaries raised by modern medicine. It is felt if we can say with some assuredness that X, Y, or Z is not a person, then our responsibility is not the same as it is to those who bear this august title.

Of course, the issue where this is most prominent is abortion. Is the fetus a human person? Supposedly, on that question hang all the law and the prophets of the morality of abortion. For if it can be shown that the fetus is not a person, as indeed I think it can be shown, then the right to the care and protection that modern medicine can provide is not due to the fetus. Indeed, the technological skill of medicine can be used to destroy such life, for its status is of no special human concern since it lacks the attribute of "personhood."

Or, for example, the issue of *when* one is a person is raised to help settle when it is morally appropriate to withdraw care from the dying. If it can be shown, for example, that a patient has moved from the status of being a person to a non-person, then it seems that many of the difficult decisions surrounding what kind and the extent of care that should be given to the dying becomes moot. For the aid that medicine can bring is directed at persons, not at the mere continuation of our bodily life. Since I will not develop it further, however, it is worth mentioning that this view assumes a rather extreme dualism between being a person and the bodily life necessary to provide the conditions for being a person (Cf Hauerwas 1974).

Or, finally, there are the issues of what kind of care should he given to defective or deformed infants in order to keep them alive. For example, Joseph Fletcher has argued that any individual who falls below the 40 I.Q. mark in a Stanford-Binet test is "questionably a person," and if you score 20 or below you are not a person (Fletcher 1972). Or Michael Tooley has argued young infants, indeed, are not "persons" and, therefore, do not bear the rights necessary to make infanticide a morally questionable practice (Tooley 1973). Whether, or what kind, of medical care should be given to children is determined by whether children are able to meet the demands of being a person. You may give them life-sustaining care, but in doing so you are acting strictly from the motive of charity since nothing obligates you to do so.

As I suggested at the first, I find all this rather odd, not because some of the conclusions reached by such reasoning may be against my own moral opinions, or because they entail practices that seem counter-intuitive (e.g., infanticide), but rather because I think this use of "person" tends to do violence to our language. For example, it is only seldom that we have occasion to think of ourselves as "persons"–when asked to identify myself, I do not think that I am a person, but I am Stanley Hauerwas, teacher, husband, father or, ultimately, a Texan. Nor do I often have the occasion to think of others as persons. I do sometimes say, "Now that Joe is one hell of a fine person," but so used, "person" carries no special status beyond the naming of a role. If I still lived in Texas, I would, as a matter of fact, never use such an expression, but rather say, "Now there is a good old boy."

Moreover, it is interesting to notice how abstract the language of person is in relation to our first-order moral language through which we live our lives and see the kind of issues I have mentioned above. For example, the reason that we do not use one man for another or society's good is not that we violate his "person," but rather because we have learned that it is destructive of the trust between us to do so. (Which is, in fact, Ramsey's real concern, as his case actually rests much more on his emphasis on the "covenant" between doctor and patient than on the status of the patient as a "person.") For example, it would surely make us hesitant to go to a doctor if we thought he might actually care for us only as means of caring for another. It should be noted, however, that in a different kind of society it might well be intelligible and trustworthy for the doctor rightly to expect that his patient be willing to undergo certain risks for the good of the society itself. I suspect that Ramsey's excessive concern to protect the patient from the demands of society through the agency of the doctor is due to living in an extraordinarily individualistic society where citizens share no good in common.

Even more artificial is the use of "person" to try to determine the moral decision in relation to abortion, death and the care of the defective new-born. For the issues surrounding whether an abortion should or should not be done seldom turn on the question of the status of the fetus. Rather, they involve why the mother does not want the pregnancy to continue, the conditions under which the pregnancy occurred, the social conditions into which the child would be born. The question of whether the fetus is or is not a person is almost a theoretical nicety in relation to the kind of questions that most abortion decisions actually involve.

Or, for example, when people are dying, we seldom decide to treat or not to treat them because they have or have not yet passed some line that makes them a person or non-person. Rather, we care or do not care for them because they are Uncle Charlie, or my father, or a good friend. In the same manner, we do not care or cease to care for a child born defective because it is or is not a person. Rather, whether or how we decide to care for such a child depends on our attitude toward the having and caring for children, our perception of our role as parents, and how medicine is seen as one form of how care is to be given to children (Hauerwas 1975). (For it may well be that we will care for such children, but this does not mean that medicine has some kind of overriding claim on being the form that such care should take.)

It might be felt that these examples assume far too easily that our common notions and stories are the primary ones for giving moral guidance in such cases. The introduction of the notion of "person" as regulatory in such matters might be an attempt to find a firmer basis than these more historically and socially contingent notions can provide. But I am suggesting that is just what the notion of "person" cannot do without seriously distorting the practices, institutions, and notions that underlay how we have learned morally to display our lives. More technically, what advocates of "personhood" have failed to show is how the notion of person works in a way of life with which we wish to identify.

Yet, we feel inextricably drawn to come up with some account that will give direction to our medical practice exactly, because we sense that our more immediate moral notions never were, or are no longer, sufficient to provide such a guide. Put concretely, we are beginning to understand how much medicine depended on the moral ethos of its society to guide how it should care for children, because we are now in a period when some people no longer think simply because a child is born to them they need regard it as their child. We will not solve this kind of dilemma by trying to say what the doctor can and cannot do in such circumstances in terms of whether the child can be understood to be a "Person" or not.

As Paul Ramsey suggests, we may have arrived at a time when we have achieved an unspeakable thing: a medical profession without a moral philosophy in a society without one either. Medicine, of course, still seems to carry the marks of a profession inasmuch as it seems to be a guardian of certain values-that is, the unconditional commitment to preserve life and health; the responsibility for justifying the patient's trust in the physician; and the autonomy of the physician in making judgments on others in the profession. But, as Alasdair Macintyre has argued, these assumed virtues can quickly be turned to vices when they lack a scheme, or, in my language, a story that depends on further beliefs about the true nature of man and our true end (MacIntyre 1975).

The language of "person" seems convenient to us, however, because we wish to assume that our medicine still rests on a consensus of moral beliefs. But I am suggesting that is exactly what is not the case and, in the absence of such a consensus, we will be much better off to simply admit that morally there are many different ways to practice medicine. We should, in other words, be willing to have our medicine as fragmented as our moral lives. I take this to be particularly important for Christians and Jews, as we have been under the illusion that we could morally expect medicine to embody our own standards, or, at least, standards that we could sympathize with. I suspect, however, that this may not be the case, for the story that determines how the virtues of medicine are to be displayed for us is quite different from the one claimed by the language of "person." (For I would not deny that advocates of "person," or the regulatory notion of medical care, are right to assume that the notion of person involves the basic libertarian values of our society. It is my claim that such values are not adequate to direct medicine in a humane and/or Christian manner.) It may be then, if we are to be honest, that we should again think of the possibility of what it might mean to practice medicine befitting our convictions as Christians or Jews. Yet, there is a heavy price to he paid for the development of such a medical practice, as it may well involve training and going to doctors whose technology is less able to cure and sustain us than current medicine provides. But, then, we must decide what is more valuable, our survival or how we choose to survive.

REFERENCES

Fletcher, Joseph (1972). 'Indicators of Humanhood.' *Hastings Center Report*. November, pp. 1-3; See also Hauerwas, Stanley. 'The Retarded and the Criteria of Human,' this volume.

Hauerwas, Stanley (1974). *Vision and Virtue: Essays in Christian Ethical Reflection*. Notre Dame, Indiana: Fides Press.

Hauerwas, Stanley (1975). 'The Demands and Limits of Care: Ethical Reflections on the Moral Dilemma of Neonatal Intensive Care.' *American Journal of Medical Science*. March-April, 1975, pp. 269-91.

MacIntyre, Alisdair (1975). 'How Virtues Become Vices: Values, Medicine, and Social Context.' *Evaluation and Explanation in the Biomedical Sciences*. Dordrecht: Reidel, pp. 97-111.

Ramsey, Paul (1970). *The Patient as Person*. New Haven: Yale University Press.

Tooley, Michael (1973). 'A Defense of Abortion and Infanticide,' in Feinberg, Joel. (Ed.), *The Problem of Abortion*. Belmont: Wadsworth Publishing Co., 51-91.

Response:
The Ground and Grammar
of Personhood

Ray Anderson, PhD, BD, BS

SUMMARY. Anderson explores the nature of personhood in the history of Christian theology. Relating this to his personal narrative of the death of his father, he challenges Hauerwas' suggestion that we should be willing to have our medical practices as fragmented as our moral lives. Taking on and enfleshing some aspects of Hauerwas' argument, Anderson suggests that giving up the language of person, in favour of each community's story and character as the primary criteria for defining and caring for others and, in the end, ourselves, is a form of semantic solipsism, if not spiritual malpractice. *[Article copies available for a fee from The Haworth Document Delivery Service: 1-800-HAWORTH. E-mail address: <docdelivery@haworthpress.com> Website: <http://www.HaworthPress.com> © 2004 by The Haworth Press, Inc. All rights reserved.]*

KEYWORDS. Person, personhood, theology, narrative, medicine

The notion of 'person,' Hauerwas suggests, is inadequate but probably also misleading and even dangerous. As a regulative notion to define the relation

Ray Anderson is Senior Professor of Theology and Ministry at Fuller Theological Seminary, Pasadena, CA 91182 USA.

[Haworth co-indexing entry note]: "Response: The Ground and Grammar of Personhood." Anderson, Ray. Co-published simultaneously in *Journal of Religion, Disability & Health* (The Haworth Pastoral Press, an imprint of The Haworth Press, Inc.) Vol. 8, No. 3/4, 2004, pp. 121-125; and: *Critical Reflections on Stanley Hauerwas' Theology of Disability: Disabling Society, Enabling Theology* (ed: John Swinton) The Haworth Pastoral Press, an imprint of The Haworth Press, Inc., 2004, pp. 121-125. Single or multiple copies of this article are available for a fee from The Haworth Document Delivery Service [1-800-HAWORTH, 9:00 a.m. - 5:00 p.m. (EST). E-mail address: docdelivery@haworthpress.com].

121

between doctor and patient the concept of person not only does violence to our language but fails to provide sufficient moral content to the practice of medicine and health care. He argues that the concept of 'person' not only suffers from abstraction by taking us out of the concrete social structure (community) and historical narrative (story) in which humans live, but can actually "distort the practices, institutions, and notions which underlay how we have learned morally to display out lives." In stating the problem his point is well taken. His illustrations are compelling. His uncle Charlie may not be a person but he is . . . well, we shall see. The pronoun 'he' can be quite elusive!

The modern use of the term 'person' in our western culture has a long history, with theological, philosophical, and moral implications. Briefly, the situation is this. The Greek word *prosopon* like the Latin *persona* originally meant a 'mask' and then the 'face.' Thus the *prosopon* or *face* is not itself the personal reality, but discloses and at the same time, hides the reality which is the essence of being human. Taking the word *hypostasis* from the Greek middle Platonic thought, which was essentially stoic, the early church theologians put a *face* on it (*prosopon*). This concept they designated as *person*. Philosophers in the Medieval period created their own language based on abstract concepts of reality to speak of human personhood. Boethius (480-524 C.E) defined person as an individuated substance possessing a rational essence. Much later, Richard of St. Victor (12th century) taught that a person is 'an incommunicable ex-sistence of an intellectual nature. While Richard, like Boethius, stressed the intellectual aspect of personhood, he used the Latin word *ex-sistentia* to indicate a quality of personal being that 'stands forth out of itself.' Thomas Aquinas (1225-1274) ignored the more dynamic view of person advanced by Richard in favor of the earlier concept of Boethius. Unfortunately, this led to a more atomistic, and even dualistic concept of human personhood which pervaded Western thought through the Reformation coming to its apex in the Enlightenment (particularly as expressed in Kant). In more recent times, this dichotomy between 'substance' and 'experience' found its way into the behavioral sciences where 'nature' tended to be viewed as behavior and 'person' as personality (Anderson 1982, pp. 5-6). The examples which Hauerwas uses to make his point are the consequence of this use of person to define the objects of concern in modern health care language and practice. Do we need a better word than 'person' or can we redeem and reclaim it for the sake of giving Uncle Charlie more than a name?

My father was dying of cancer and lapsed into a partial coma at which time the family was summoned to his bedside in his own home. At first, he seemed aware of our conversation, indicated by movements of his hands, but unable to speak. Later in the day, the coma became more complete, he no longer was able to make any movements. Holding his hand and monitoring his heartbeat,

I felt the final shudder of the heart muscle and the last heart beat. "He is gone," said my brother. Really, I thought? His flesh was still warm, there were minor contractions of the muscles. His sister gently closed his eyes and took two coins to place over his eyelids. Tying a cloth around his head to close his gaping mouth, she restored his face, his dignity, and his humanity. Within an hour the family physician came, determined that his heart had indeed stopped, turned to us and said, "He is gone, he is dead." Leaving as efficiently as he came, we were left to ponder the mystery of the presence (and apparent departure) of a father, husband, and brother.

In retrospect, I continue to ponder the significance of the pronoun 'he.' To say of my father, 'he is gone' seemed premature as the reality to which the pronoun 'he' referred was no different at that moment then it was twenty-four hours (or twenty-four years) earlier. At the funeral service his pastor comforted the family by saying of our father, 'He is now with the Lord.' By this time it had become quite clear that the pronoun 'he' had become quite internalized in our minds and in our faith. That was 53 years ago. Only two years ago, walking with my children through the rural cemetery marking out the various tomb stones, I came to one and said, 'This is my father's, this is where he is buried.'

Now I know for sure that the elusive pronoun 'he' has become separated from that reality to which I referred not only during my father's active life, but even more during the final days and hours which he was unable to speak and respond. So, what is the reality to which the personal pronoun 'he' refers? Was it never more than some internalized mental or emotional construct in the subject who thought and spoke it? Was there ever any objective reality which gave the pronoun its meaning?

Common sense would quickly reject the notion that in our ordinary lives the words 'he' or 'she' are only subjective constructs of our minds or, at the most, functional terms by which we differentiate between one and another. Hauerwas has it right when he says that 'My uncle Charlie is not much of a person but he is still my uncle Charlie.' At the end, my father was not able to make much of a response, but he was still my father.

What seems to be at stake in this discussion is not so much a philosophy of personhood as it is the relation of language itself to being. "We do not use language," Martin Heidegger liked to say, "but language uses us. Language is the house of being" Heideggar (1971). Thomas Torrance argues that our modern age suffers from a separation of language from being. We cannot use words to define the relation between words and the objective reality which words signify. At the same time we must assume that there is such a relation, otherwise we are cut off from reality and experience what he calls the 'culture split' between explanation (*erklären*) and understanding (*verstehen*) (Torrance 1965, pp. 18-20).

Throughout his life, I would have said that my father was a person. In the ordinary sense of the word we are all persons. At the same time, as Torrance reminds us, the relation of the word 'person' to that which it signifies can be a real relation but at the same time ambiguous and tenuous. I would argue that the very ambiguity which lies between the pronoun 'she' and the person that my daughter is, for example, creates the moral and spiritual space in which we live by intention, trust, and responsibility. I agree with Hauerwas that the moral imperative which binds one person to another is not a deontological ethical duty in the Kantian sense. At the same time, I want to argue that what anchors the moral sense in caring for persons under extreme and difficult conditions is the substantive reality of persons and not merely a 'community' of ethical character and concern such as I read Hauerwas advocating.

The grammar of personhood is woven into the biblical tradition. David muses on his own existence as the object of divine care and concern, even in his prenatal state. 'For it was you who formed my inward parts; you knit me together in my mother's womb. . . . My frame was not hidden from you when I was being made in secret' (Psalm 119: 13, 15). David internalizes his existence as a person by using the personal form of self-reference–my, me, I. This is the grammar of personhood but it is also grounded not only in divine intentionality but in concrete fetal existence. In a remarkable passage for its eschatological hope, David responds to the tragic death of his son by saying, "I shall go to him, but he will not return to me" (2 Samuel 12:23). Here again we encounter the elusive pronoun 'he.' This, of course, is the language and grammar of faith. But it is the grammar of personhood as well. Despite the ambiguous and tenuous existence of persons under the conditions of distress and mortality, by using the term person we lift ourselves and others out of the indiscriminate and impersonal fate of mere creaturely being, enter into the ambiguous space to consecrate and connect with personal being as the ground of our own existence and the gift of others.

Martin Buber has reminded us that impersonal objects and concepts (it) cannot call forth and authenticate the personal reality of 'I.' Only another 'thou' can call forth and affirm the 'I' (Buber 1970). To say 'me' as a form of self reference is intended to denote personal being–that I am a person! The relation between the word 'me' and the person that I really am is both ambiguous and tenuous. I live in that space with moral and spiritual intentionality and integrity. I expect others who refer to me as 'he' to hold me accountable for being who I am in the same way that I hold those whom I call he or she accountable for being who they really are. Cannot we say that we are persons in this way?

In using the word 'person' in his sense I agree that the term is semantically ambiguous but morally significant. In the first few weeks of a pregnancy my wife suffered a miscarriage. Was this the death of a person? Not to our way of thinking. To use the term person to speak of embryonic tissue presses the semantical connection between the word and that which it signifies beyond its capacity to bear meaning. At the same time, the very ambiguity calls for sensitivity and responsibility for a developmental process through which personhood emerges, sometimes precariously premature and usually punctually when due. At any point when personhood appears to be viable, that viable life demands personal attention and moral concern. With a sonogram which reveals the sex of a fetus the pronoun he or she becomes semantically significant, even though precarious. There is no certainty that personhood will survive the birth process and, correspondingly, there is no certainty as to when personhood departs in the dying process. The ambiguity, I suggest is not in regard to *who* a person is, but rather *what* we mean when we use the term. Those who become patients due to physical, emotional or mental distress, as well as those who suffer with some form of disability, have no doubts as to *who* they are and we should have no doubt as to *how* we interact with and treat them. The grammar of human personhood is grounded in those whom we call persons. To paraphrase, Shakespeare, a person by any other name, is still a person!

In the end, I worry about Hauerwas' conclusion that we should be as willing to have medical practice as fragmented as our moral lives. Giving up the language of person, in favor of each community's story and character as the primary criteria for defining and caring for others and, in the end, ourselves, is a form of semantic solipsism if not spiritual malpractice. If I were to suggest a revision of the title of Hauerwas' essay it would be: *Every Patient is a Person, and My Uncle Charlie is a Person Too!*

REFERENCES

Anderson, Ray S. (1982). *On Being Human: Essays in Theological Anthropology*. Grand Rapids: Eerdmans.
Buber, Martin. (1970). *I and Thou*. Edinburgh: T & T Clark.
Heidegger, M. (1971). *On the Way to Language*. New York: Harper and Row.
Torrance, Thomas F. (1965). *Theology in Reconstruction*. Grand Rapids: Eerdmans.

Chapter 7

The Retarded
and the Criteria for the Human

Stanley Hauerwas, PhD

[From *Truthfulness and Tragedy: Further investigations into Christian ethics* (1977, pp. 156-163)]. Reprinted with permission.

SUMMARY. The criteria for what is understood as authentic 'humanhood' have been much discussed in contemporary bioethics. Many of the 'traditional' arguments for the essence of humanness necessarily exclude people with developmental disabilities. Such definitions can easily lead to treatment which is inhumane. Hauerwas critque's the criteria for humanness arguing that the conditions of being human form a far too complex pattern ever to be reduced to 'criteria.' To be human is to be open to the call of what we are not, and there is therefore no chance that our humanity will be enhanced by excluding from our ranks those who we do not understand as 'we.'

KEYWORDS. Humanness, personhood, bioethics, criteria for being human

---

[Haworth co-indexing entry note]: "The Retarded and the Criteria for the Human." Hauerwas, Stanley. Co-published simultaneously in *Journal of Religion, Disability & Health* (The Haworth Pastoral Press, an imprint of The Haworth Press, Inc.) Vol. 8, No. 3/4, 2004, pp. 127-134; and: *Critical Reflections on Stanley Hauerwas' Theology of Disability: Disabling Society, Enabling Theology* (ed: John Swinton) The Haworth Pastoral Press, an imprint of The Haworth Press, Inc., 2004, pp. 127-134. Single or multiple copies of this article are available for a fee from The Haworth Document Delivery Service [1-800-HAWORTH, 9:00 a.m. - 5:00 p.m. (EST). E-mail address: docdelivery@haworthpress.com].

CRITERIA OF THE HUMAN IN RECENT ETHICS

It is often argued that the evaluation of the development and application of new biomedical technology depends on the view one has of man. The degree one thinks man is different from other animals and in what that difference consists seems to be crucial for such issues as the prolongation of life, the limits or uses of behavior modification, and the permissibility of human experimentation. Even though the centrality of our view of man for such decisions seems obvious, how the "distinctively human" is to be understood and used is a matter of controversy. This difficulty may be an indication that there is something morally askew about the general methodological assumption that criteria for the human are required for the work of bioethies to advance. For this assumption makes us forget how inappropriate it is for the preservation of our humanity to justify the exclusion of some men from human care and concern on grounds that they fail to meet such "criteria." The appropriate moral context for raising the question of the "essentially" human should not be an attempt to determine if some men are or are not human, but rather what we must be if we are to preserve and enhance what humanity we have. In other words the question of the criteria of the human should not be raised about others but only about ourselves.

Many raise the question of the "distinctively" human in an attempt to place some limits on what they perceive as the dehumanizing potential of biomedical technology. For example, they argue that we should not try to create "better humans" through positive genetic manipulation, as these procedures violate man's dignity and capacity for self-determination. For example in *Chicago Studies* (Fall, 1972), William May argues that we should not do what we can do because:

> man does differ, and differs radically in kind from other animals and that this difference is rooted in his capacity for conceptual thought, propositional speech, and self-determination. It is a difference, moreover, implicitly recognized by the majority of contemporary scientists and is affirmed in a very striking way in a comment made by Willard Gaylin, MD, professor of psychiatry and law at Columbia University, when he wrote: "The human being is the only species capable of systematically altering its normal biological system by use of its equally normal intellectual capacity."

It is unclear, however, if this kind of appeal to the "distinctively" human is sufficient to place limitations on our technological powers. For example, many justify greater scientific manipulation by appealing to similar conceptions of man as the being open to constant self-modification through our capacity for self-determination.

Inhumane Treatment

Both sides of this debate fail to notice that their understanding of "distinctively" human embodies values that warrant inhumane treatment toward some in our society because they do not comply with such criteria. In their enthusiasm to assert the dignity of man as either enhanced or destroyed by technology, they formulate criteria of the human that appear in our cultural context as an *ideology* for the strong. For example, such criteria clearly embody our assumption that mans rational and cognitive ability is what makes us human. Yet this belief is the basis for the inhumane treatment and care our society provides for the retarded, as we assume such people are fundamentally other than and foreign to the human community. Our responsibility to them extends to keeping them alive, but humanizing care beyond securing their survival is simply not warranted since they lack the essential conditions to claim the care provided for those that are "fully human." Such treatment tragically becomes a self-fulfilling prophecy as we dehumanize them through impersonal and institutional cruelty or, in some ways even more destructive, the smothering care of pity. Not to be able to think as we think, to talk as we talk, or to do as we do is to forfeit ones right to be treated with respect due to another human.

The presence of the retarded serves as a significant test case for any attempt to determine the "distinctively" human. For surely any criteria of the human that would justify less than human care for the retarded on the grounds that they fall outside the purview of our species is morally suspect. The perverse effects of such a limited sense of the human can be seen not only in the kind of care we provide for many of the retarded in our society but with the stigma we associate with retardation. To describe someone as retarded is not a technical decision based on neutral scientific data and analysis: The criteria that determine retardation have less to do with the "weakness" of the retarded than with the complexity of the demands of our society as well as our tolerance of deviation. In a society already so inhumane, we can ill afford to enshrine our inhumanity in formal criteria that putatively are presented to prevent technology's encroachment on the "essentially" human.

This argument can he made in a less dramatic way by pointing out that the criteria of the distinctively human are not simply a list of empirical characteristics. The notion of the human is a conceptualization that makes meaningful or better intelligible why we associate certain empirical features with being human at all. In other words the evidence for our particular understanding of the human is dependent on prior conceptual and normative commitments that must be justified philosophically and ethically, since it cannot be assumed that the "empirical" conditions we have learned to associate with being man are necessary to the human conceptually and normatively understood. As James Gustafson has said, "A prejudgment about what is and is not truly human probably lurks in the judgment about what data to use in describing the human." Therefore, to raise the question of the criteria of the human is not first an empirical question, but a conceptual-moral claim about how the nature of man should be understood. We wrongly assume that what our eyes perceive as "normal" is what we should morally understand men to be qua human. The presence of the retarded helps us feel the oddness and the problematic nature of this assumption and its attendant ethical implications.

Fletcher's Position

The significance of this argument can be illustrated by contrasting it with Joseph Fletcher's attempt to provide the biomedical decision maker with a profile of the human in operational terms (Fletcher 1972). Fletcher's "profile" includes fifteen positive and five negative propositions that are meant to provide necessary and sufficient grounds for attributing the status of human to another. To be man we must be capable of self-awareness, self-control, have a sense of time, futurity and past, be capable of relating to others, show concern for others, be able to communicate, exert control over our existence, be curious, be open to changes, have a proper balance of rationality and feeling, and have a unique identity. Negatively, men are not any of the following: anti-artificial, essentially parents, sexual, worshipers, or a bundle of rights. I am sure each of us will have our special problem with one or more of these criteria, especially as some seem to make recommendations about how to be a good or mature man rather than the minimal conditions necessary to be a man. However, it is not my purpose to try to evaluate each of these "criteria" separately, as I am interested in trying to make a more general point concerning the vagueness of this list. Fletcher claims to have developed a list of "operational" criteria that are empirically specifiable, but all the conditions listed have only the vaguest empirical correlates. For example, what "empirical" signs could be given as a necessary warrant to demonstrate that someone had control over himself that would be useful to the doctor?

The issue is complicated by Fletcher's failure to distinguish between criteria that are necessary and those that are sufficient to determine the human. For example, if a criterion such as having a proper balance between rationality and feeling is a necessary condition for being human, then I suspect some of us are in perpetual peril of losing our status as humans. However, Fletcher does identify minimal intelligence provided by the neo-cortical function as *the* necessary empirical condition on which all these other characteristics depend. "In a way," he says, "this is the cardinal indicator, the one all the others are hinged upon. Before cerebration is in play, or with its end, in the absence of the synthesizing function of the cerebral cortex, the *person* is nonexistent. Such individuals are objects but not subjects" (Fletcher 1972, p. 3). Fletcher's emphasis on this aspect of our physiology rests on his assumption that to be human is to be rational, or in his language, "*Homo* is indeed *sapiens*, in order to be *homo*. *The ratio*, in another turn of speech, is what makes a person of the *vita*. Mere biological life, before minimal intelligence is achieved or after it is lost irretrievably, is without personal status" (Fletcher 1972, p. 1).

Thus, for Fletcher any individual who falls below the I.Q. 40 mark in a Stanford-Binet test is "questionably a person," and if you score 20 or below you are not a person.

Before raising the more substantive issues about Fletchers position, there are some empirical issues that should be considered. It is interesting that Fletcher places such great faith in the Stanford-Binet test, since it is extremely unclear what such a test measures (even psychologists are not all sure what intelligence involves or how the Stanford-Binet relates to intelligence). Therefore, even on empirical grounds it is not clear that the one operational criterion Fletcher gives to mark off the human is anything less than arbitrary. More troublesome than this is what empirical features Fletcher would associate with the absence of neo-cortical function, since it could involve anything from the loss of an EEG to the beginnings of senility. Fletcher seems to base his position in this respect on the assumption that activities such as instrumental learning and cognition reside entirely in the neo-cortex, but this has not yet been decisively established. Of course, no one would wish to deny the significance of the neo-cortex for our behavior, yet we should at least be aware that the identification of brain and mind is fraught with philosophical and empirical difficulties. Recent research suggests that we must be careful how we draw the distinction between body and mind, since it may be that our spirit and individuality is more dependent on "mere biological processes" than we had thought.

Purpose of Criteria

More substantively it can be asked what purpose Fletcher's criteria are to serve–that is, what conclusions should be drawn from them and what tasks should we try to perform with them? They seem to lend themselves to an interpretation that would exclude many that are now receiving care as human beings. Should we cease trying to obtain better living and learning conditions for the profoundly and moderately retarded? What should be done with the elderly who are no longer able to meet the criteria of being members of the Pepsi-generation? Should we cease developing resources for the care of those whose intelligence is not up to coping with our modern society because they place a drain on our resources while not contributing to the services or artifacts of our civilization?

The "profile" of man does not, I suspect, provide operational criteria any doctor would recognize, but it is rather a statement of the working assumptions about the value of human life that are alive in our culture. The strong stress on the value of intelligence as the necessary condition for all human activity faithfully mirrors the loyalties of our society. Intelligence, however, is not an end in itself, nor is our ability to reason sufficient to make us human if being human has anything to do with being humane. To assert such criteria as necessary to being human separated from the values and community for which they exist is to risk perversions we can scarcely afford in a world that already condemns some children to a miserable existence because they cannot exercise "problem-solving" intelligence. We fail to notice that such criteria are really goals through which we manipulate and destroy some for the good of the "normal." The important moral question is not whether the retarded meet or should meet "criteria of the human" we have established, but whether we do not become inhuman by being concerned with such judgements rather than providing the retarded with respect and care.

Our society's high value of rationality tends to make us forget that our ability to think cannot be separated from our nature as social beings. As G.H. Mead taught, we would never be able to distinguish the "me" and the "not me," the bedrock of awareness and reason, if we were not graced with the presence of the other. This descriptive point provides the basis for the more substantive ethical claim that our capacity to reason rightly is a correlative of our ability to regard others with respect. The use of the criterion of intelligence to warrant the exclusion of those that repel and think differently from us is to cut off the moral basis of our ability to be rational at all. Put in more traditional terminology, our rational ability is not the prior principle of our moral activity, for we are able to reason because we are fundamentally social beings. To emphasize our rational ability separated from its social-moral context is to intellectualize arbitrarily the power of cognition and language.

Being Human

To be a man is to be able to perceive and respond to other men with recognition of care. It is unclear to me what empirical criteria are correlative of this understanding of man since the forms of response are rich and varied. That we need to develop some empirical rules of thumb to check our arbitrariness in some of the hard cases occasioned by our increased technological skill is not in question. As Eric Cassell suggests, "The function of morality in medicine is no longer simply to protect the weak and the sick from indifference or venality, but to protect them also from mercy grown overwhelming by technological advance." However, the development of such rules of thumb must be developed with the kind of exactness that such cases entail, rather than with the generality that opens them to the perversion of justifying our uncaring towards those who do not fit our current standards of "fully human."

In this respect, I think a strong cautionary note needs to be interjected about developing criteria of the human that will somehow relieve us of the hard choices that we are confronting in modern medicine. For criteria that are sufficient for all the kinds of cases we confront will be so vague that their concrete implications will be ambiguous at best. Even if you try to make such criteria more operational for the doctor by tying them to empirical characteristics, it is by no means clear that the moral questions involved in many of these cases will be any more resolvable. For, even though such criteria may help you decide that this life is not "fully human," the question of whether care should be given still remains. I suspect that we are human exactly to the extent we can reach out and provide care for those who have no "right" to it. Put more concretely, as important as criteria are to inform decisions, we cannot make them do all the work of ethical judgment and argument for all cases, since no criterion is going to relieve, or should make less troublesome, the burden of deciding to operate to save the life of a severely retarded child. To try to substitute "impersonal criteria" for what should be the moral agony of such decisions is already to sacrifice more of our humanity than we can stand.

Finally, I think we should feel more the oddness of trying to determine this or that as the criterion that makes us human. The conditions of being human form a far too complex pattern to ever be reduced to something like "criteria." Too quick appeals to the mystery of being human can be but excuses for cloudy and sloppy thinking that attempts to evade some of the hard issues we are confronting, but they may also be profound responses to the human sense that ultimately we are not our own creators. To be a man is to be open to the call of what we are not, and there is, therefore, no chance that our humanity will be enhanced by excluding from our ranks those who do not understand as we. We must therefore approach the attempt to develop criteria of the human with the humility that recognizes that we would be less than human if we did not recognize that there are limits to what can be brought under our control.

REFERENCES

Fletcher, Joseph (1972). 'Indicators of Humanhood: A Tentative Profile of Man.' *Hastings Center Report.* Volume 2, Number 5, November.
May, William. *Chicago Studies* (Fall, 1972). (Full reference missing from original text).

EDITOR'S NOTE

It will be noted that references from Gustafson, Mead, and Cassel are not included in the essay. This is due to their absence from the original text.

Chapter 8

Suffering, Medical Ethics, and the Retarded Child

Stanley Hauerwas, PhD

[From *Truthfulness and Tragedy: Further investigations into Christian ethics* (1977, pp. 164-168)]. Reprinted with permission.

SUMMARY. Hauerwas explores the nature of suffering as the term is applied to the lives of people with developmental disabilities. He asks the question "whose suffering is it that is relieved by such medical technologies as amniocentesis?" Is it the suffering of the child? Or is it the suffering of the family or even the wider society? Such questions raise major moral issues relating to medicine and the type of society that we hope to bring about. Hauerwas presents a framework within which we can wrestle with these questions and begin to understand the nature and purpose of suffering.

[Haworth co-indexing entry note]: "Suffering, Medical Ethics, and the Retarded Child." Hauerwas, Stanley. Co-published simultaneously in *Journal of Religion, Disability & Health* (The Haworth Pastoral Press, an imprint of The Haworth Press, Inc.) Vol. 8, No. 3/4, 2004, pp. 135-140; and: *Critical Reflections on Stanley Hauerwas' Theology of Disability: Disabling Society, Enabling Theology* (ed: John Swinton) The Haworth Pastoral Press, an imprint of The Haworth Press, Inc., 2004, pp. 135-140. Single or multiple copies of this article are available for a fee from The Haworth Document Delivery Service [1-800-HAWORTH, 9:00 a.m. - 5:00 p.m. (EST). E-mail address: docdelivery@haworthpress.com].

http://www.haworthpress.com/web/JRDH
Digital Object Identifier: 10.1300/J095v8n03_16

KEYWORDS. Suffering, developmental disability, community, bioethics

Certain areas of contemporary medicine are important for medical ethics because they raise in a particularly intense and fruitful form issues that cut across the general practice of medicine. For instance, the development of amniocentesis and various procedures for keeping alive children previously considered hopelessly ill have made fetal care and neonatology very interesting for ethical reflection. The cases confronted in these areas reveal the simplistic character of many moral guidelines which have been generally accepted in medical practice. The doctor, for example, has traditionally assumed he should always act to relieve suffering. But it is becoming increasingly apparent that such a principle is simply not sufficient for dealing with issues like whether retarded children should be born or cared for. Or put more strongly, we are learning that the principle enjoining the doctor always to relieve suffering, when unqualifiedly accepted, has implications which are anything but life-enhancing.

Let me illustrate these remarks by discussing some cases that are prevalent today in fetal and neonatal medicine. When a woman undergoes amniocentesis and discovers that the fetus has Downs Syndrome, a common conclusion is that the fetus should be aborted. The decision to abort is often justified as necessary to spare such children and their families a life of suffering, embarrassment and discrimination. Thus the doctor's assumption that he should always act to relieve suffering seems to support such a decision. But upon reflection this is an odd application, for traditionally the principle to relieve suffering has been understood as enhancing life. The transformation of the principle in this context to one of life-denial demonstrates how quickly abstract principles can be reinterpreted when they become divorced from their customary uses.

This kind of problem indicates the complexity involved in reflection on medical ethics. The renewed interest in medical ethics is encouraging, but we cannot assume this will result in the development of clear and unambiguous guidelines for medical practice. For principles are only summary statements of the values and inherited moral wisdom shared by the community or profession about the nature of human existence. Useful though principles are, they easily can be and are divorced from the original insights that gave them substance, forming ideologies for quite a different set of practices. This is why the moral commitments doctors often embody in practice are frequently more substantive than the principles they explicitly invoke. The problem is, however, that no practice can be sustained which is not properly mirrored in language and ritual. Probably one reason why medical ethics is becoming important is the necessity doctors are feeling to learn the moral language of their art. Inability to articulate the language is finally failure to practice medicine morally.

Doctor's adherence to the principle of alleviating suffering provides a good illustration of why they must understand how the principle works in relation to other basic commitments in medical practice, as well as knowing what the principle itself means. Although doctors in the past have claimed to act as if the obligation to relieve suffering were unqualified, in actual practice the principle functioned as a limited obligation. It has always been regarded legitimate to ask patients to endure limited forms of pain and suffering in order to regain health. Thus the principle requiring the doctor to alleviate suffering has been, in fact, morally qualified by the physicians conception of health and the therapy necessary to achieve it.

The medical profession has generally assumed that "health" should be understood primarily as the normal functioning of the physical and physiological aspects of our being. "Psychological" considerations have been taken into account insofar as they have a bearing on the patient's physical condition. By assuming that a retarded child ought to be aborted to spare it and the family suffering, however, the doctor is accepting an immensely broadened meaning of "suffering" and "pain." (Not to mention that in such circumstances the difficult problem of *who is the patient* is raised!) What the retarded child and its family are now to be spared are the difficulties occasioned by an indifferent and cruel society which rejects those who fail to meet its requirements for "normality." That is a far cry from the traditional concept of the suffering which the physician is pledged to alleviate. It is questionable whether medicine can accept this enlarged sense of relieving "suffering" without being perverted. For, in contemporary society, it is not only retarded persons who face the suffering which comes from embarrassing, annoying, frightening, or threatening those who regard themselves and their way of life as "normal." If the medical profession is willing to serve a certain societal ethos in relation to those diagnosed as retarded, why should it not use its technical power against other groups which deviate from the society's accepted standards? A doctor's commitment to alleviate suffering can readily be deflected and co-opted for highly questionable purposes in a society which identifies suffering with psychological and economic discomfort. It is all too easy to fail to notice that in the name of sparing others suffering one must justify a Promethean presumption to control and determine their very existence. The greatest evils are, of course, always perpetrated on others in the name of "their own good." Viewed in this perspective, a doctor's traditional commitment to the physical appears as a substantial moral value which protects his art from the arbitrariness of societal norms.

The care of the retarded child, however, is perhaps not the hardest one for exploring the limits of the principle of the alleviation of suffering and the practice associated with it. Cases of children born with grave abnormalities raise the issue in a different and perhaps more intense form. For it is possible to have a prognosis for these children which gives accurate information regarding the physical suffering they will undergo for what may be at best only a few years of life. It seems a natural and human question to ask why we should not be willing to let such children die in order to spare them this futile agony.

A first response to such a question might be to deny that there is any one principle which can provide an answer to it. Principles, even understood as rules of thumb, tend to assume an independent existence. When they are too consistently applied, they generally result in inhumanity. For the principle gives us an illusion of objectivity and impartiality in an area where we best not forget we are fallible and often arbitrary beings. Letting one severely deformed infant die to relieve suffering should not establish a rule for all subsequent cases; such a rule would only close off life-giving opportunities for the future. I suspect many doctors working in neonatal wards tend to preserve the distinction between "letting die" and "putting to death" because they fear the latter description would require giving general reasons for their action which might limit their choice for future cases. The distinction between "letting die" and "putting to death" relies heavily on the assumption that in such cases there is a real difference between refraining from giving care and acting to end a life. The doctor knows well, however, that by "refraining" to give care he is putting the child to death. He refuses to describe it as such because as a doctor he fears the implications such a description might have for the care of future patients. This may suggest that even though in certain circumstances acting to put to death is not descriptively easily distinguished from refraining to act. There are good moral reasons to maintain the distinction in order to enforce the doctor's commitment to save life. If this is the case, however, it is extremely important that we develop criteria for the careful use of the distinction.

It is unhappily true that for many children the most humane response is to protect them from a mercy grown overwhelming by technological advances that can sustain their life beyond any good end. However, in such cases we must be careful to be clear whose suffering we are most concerned to end, the patient's physical and mental pain, or our pain occasioned by having to be next to a patient we cannot relieve. We should never overlook the threat we feel at having to be near those who suffer, even if it is the suffering or assumed future suffering of a new-born. In such circumstances our very humanity can be transformed into inhumanity as we recoil in hate against the other for revealing our helplessness. Our very humanity can force us to dehumanize the sufferer, because he reminds us too strongly of the fragility of the human condition. Such dehumanization is but the first step toward elimination.

Ironically, in order to spare the other person suffering, we may be willing literally to deny him existence. But why should we assume that existence is only valuable when it is free from suffering? Why should we assume that we should always try to spare the other suffering when we know that often the good we do comes only because we were willing to endure pain? It is hard to calculate the importance of these questions for medical practice. If we assume that we ought always to deal with suffering by elimination, then there is nothing that can force the imagination to develop new forms of care and cure.

Medicine advances because doctors and others in helping professions have been willing to allow others to endure pain. By our willingness to stand in the presence of such pain we create the conditions that impel the imagination to explore yet unthought forms of care. Not to be willing to witness suffering makes it too easy to forget that the patient and not the disease is the object of the doctor's care. Such a tendency can be illustrated in the way we refer to retarded people as "retardates" or "mongoloids," thereby seeing abstractions rather than individuals afflicted with Downs Syndrome. When we class them as "mongoloids," we forget that a person is more than a disease; and this may lead to the assumption that in trying to eliminate such diseases it is incidental if we must also eliminate the person. Progress toward better care for persons so afflicted will be made, however, if we do not forget that these are people–suffering people to be sure–who claim our attention and care even if we cannot "cure" their affliction or protect them against suffering. The task of the doctor is not simply to alleviate suffering. He must stand before those who suffer without denying their being. The doctor's task is to provide care even when such care may involve the patient in suffering. Of course, there are limits to the ability of doctors to act in this fashion. Cases where parents refuse to allow life-saving surgery on their retarded or deformed children are the most dramatic instances of this kind of problem. It may be that in the absence of societal support for such children we cannot argue that the parents or the doctors have an obligation to perform surgery in such circumstances.

However, what is not clear about such cases is why the parents have been relieved from the burden of care for the child until it dies. Doctors have no responsibility to watch the child die in the name of sparing the parents suffering; nor should they accept such responsibility, for otherwise the parents have no sense of the full reality of the decision they have made. The doctor's willingness to protect the parents from the death of these children unwittingly supports a societal ethos that would eliminate rather than care for those that cause us discomfort. It may seem excessively cruel to ask parents who decide not to give a retarded child care to take it home, but otherwise the medical profession too easily protects our society from the knowledge that we do not care to protect the life of these children.

It is perhaps necessary in conclusion to forestall misunderstanding. I am not suggesting that suffering should be sought for its own sake; or that suffering should be accepted as a way of becoming good. I have no sympathy for some religious and philosophical traditions that make suffering an inherent good. Rather, I am trying to suggest that though suffering is not to be sought, neither must we assume it should always be avoided. Often we achieve the good only because we are willing to endure in ourselves and others an existence of suffering and pain.

A Response to Chapters Seven and Eight: Retarded Children or Retarded Ethics?

Christopher Newell, PhD

SUMMARY. Newell responds to the essays presented in chapters seven and eight. The way in which disability removes dignity and claims to personhood in accounts of contemporary ethics is explored in contemplating Hauerwas' perceptive work, suggesting he led the way in understanding this phenomenon. Yet, for all the value of his insights, it is suggested we need an account of medical ethics, and bioethics in general, which moves beyond talking about disability to being informed by, and commencing with, the narratives of people with disability. *[Article copies available for a fee from The Haworth Document Delivery Service: 1-800-HAWORTH. E-mail address: <docdelivery@haworthpress.com> Website: <http://www.HaworthPress.com> © 2004 by The Haworth Press, Inc. All rights reserved.]*

KEYWORDS. Children, disability, ethics, utilitarianism, theology, humanness

I come to the work of Stanley Hauerwas as a person with disability. Many years of institutional care and professionals talking *about* me and my very different account of ethics, has helped shape my personal approach to teaching and

[Haworth co-indexing entry note]: "A Response to Chapters Seven and Eight: Retarded Children or Retarded Ethics?". Newell, Christopher. Co-published simultaneously in *Journal of Religion, Disability & Health* (The Haworth Pastoral Press, an imprint of The Haworth Press, Inc.) Vol. 8, No. 3/4, 2004, pp. 141-147; and: *Critical Reflections on Stanley Hauerwas' Theology of Disability: Disabling Society, Enabling Theology* (ed: John Swinton) The Haworth Pastoral Press, an imprint of The Haworth Press, Inc., 2004, pp. 141-147. Single or multiple copies of this article are available for a fee from The Haworth Document Delivery Service [1-800-HAWORTH, 9:00 a.m. - 5:00 p.m. (EST). E-mail address: docdelivery@haworthpress.com].

practicing ethics. Accordingly, I approach the subject of theological ethics from a different, but complementary, perspective to that of Professor Hauerwas. My task in this essay is to begin to explore where these two perspectives intersect and reflect on the implications of such a dialogue. Let me begin by sharing some of my own experiences in teaching ethics to undergraduate medical students.

AN EXERCISE IN PRACTICAL ETHICS

One of the first concepts that I explore in my Medical Ethics lectures for these emerging medical practitioners is the notion of humanness, as espoused by Joseph Fletcher and critiqued by Stanley Hauerwas. There is little better way of critically examining Fletcher's criteria than to take someone regarded as a "normal" (i.e., non-disabled) member of the moral community and strip that person of the various attributes which Fletcher defines as being important for humanness.

Step 1

Take a "volunteer" first year medical student, and separate him or her from their peers. A "volunteer" is defined as anyone unlucky enough to sit in the front row of the lecture theatre!

Step 2

With a "flick of one's magical fingers" transform the student (a person) into an objectified *other* (a non-person). The essence of the process is as follows:

a. Talk about the student as if he was not a party to what was going on.
b. Provide him/her with a new identity–*disabled*.
c. Slowly strip away the various attributes which Fletcher defines as being important, whilst at the same time making similar collective discoveries with regard to the difficulties and arbitrariness of our notions of humanness.
d. Remove the student's ability to communicate, reason, contribute to society and so forth.
e. As the disabilities "grow" we discuss whether the student should be put out of his or her suffering (remembering to avoid eye contact with the student at all times in order that your ethical reflection truly resembles dislocated, depersonalized academic medical ethics!)–asking if it is their suffering or ours to which the majority are responding. Remember to take seriously Hauerwas' insight that: "In order to spare the other persons suffering we may be willing literally to deny him existence. But

why should we assume that existence is only valuable when it is free of suffering?"

This simple exercise helps to show the importance of Stanley Hauerwas' thinking in the two essays which were presented previously. When ethics are done *on* people rather than *with* them, all sorts of unpleasant things can happen.

The Rise of "Retarded" Ethics

It would be easy for us to dismiss Hauerwas' work as being dated, since rarely do we talk of "the retarded" these days. Yet, whilst our language may have changed a bit, the social prejudices found in this language remain. Indeed they are often cloaked in the guise of "therapy" as we remove people with disabilities from the moral community, and justify our actions with consequentialist accounts of ethics which have gained growing popularity. If in doubt, consider the rise in popularity of the work of such thinkers as Peter Singer. Despite the protests of people with disabilities around the world Singer adopts a utilitarian stance of classic dimensions, whereby ethics, and our conduct, are to be directed by the calculation of the greatest good for the greatest number, with 'good' being understood primarily in relation to pleasure or the absence of pain. A consistent implication of his ethics is that people with disability, as a minority, are inevitably, indeed inherently, disadvantaged by such accounts. In a variety of books and articles he has argued that, as one article puts it well, "Killing isn't always wrong," a position which advocates the moral correctness of infanticide on the grounds of disability (Singer, 1995). Elsewhere he has argued that some people with "mental retardation" have such impairment that they have lesser claim to life than some animals:

> So should we accept the premise that every human being has a right to life? We may do so, but only if we bear in mind that by 'human being' here we refer to those beings who have the mental qualities which general distinguish members of our species from members of other species. (Singer et al., 1990, p. 70)

I have yet to meet a thoroughgoing utilitarian who has significant disability–such a person would vanish in a puff of logic given the impact of such a position on members of minority groups. Further, Singer (in conjunction with Kuhse) locate the problem in terms of impaired bodies and minds rather than the social system. For example, in their book *Should the Baby Live? The Problem of Handicapped Infants* (Kuhse & Singer, 1985), the "problem" of Down's syndrome is located firmly within the body of the child. The phrasing of their subtitle says it all. Such work locates the problem in terms of retarded children. Hauerwas on the other hand, in line with the work of many contemporary scholars with disabilities points to fundamentally retarded and limited accounts of ethics as the locus of the problem. In the aforementioned book, Singer and Kuhse explore the challenges of disability in infants, especially neonates, concluding that it is ethical within the first twenty-eight days of life to kill children considered, by them, to be unworthy of life. They conclude in stark terms: "We think that some infants with severe disabilities should be killed" (Kuhse & Singer, 1985: 173). Yet, as with much work in medical ethics, they fail to recognize that society handicaps people in terms of structures and attitudes, with norms that mean impairment is significant rather than of minor impact (see Oliver, 1996: 143; Davis, 1989).

Disability as Suffering?

Every day as I practice as an ethicist, work as an Anglican priest, and seek to accompany people on the journey of life I become more and more aware of the epistemological significance of my experience of disability and suffering and the ways in which it shapes and underpins my practice and my teaching. The world of disability sees things very differently from the world of the able-bodied. Similarly, those commonly referred to as "retarded" or who, like my unwitting volunteer student, lack communication, have much to teach us. The insidious practice and indeed the technological determinism alluded to by Hauerwas has become all pervasive. Increasingly, those of us who live with disability see that in the guise of "therapy," "medical advance," and "progress," our very existence and legitimacy is questioned. Hauerwas is truly prophetic when he writes: "A doctor's commitment to alleviate suffering can readily be deflected and co-opted for highly questionable purposes in a society which identifies suffering with psychological and economic discomfort. . . . The greatest evils are, of course, always perpetuated on others in the name of "their own good."

Such a perspective is particularly important when we look at the way in which many justifications for interventions in the life-cycle from screening, genetic screening, through reproductive and cloning technology to euthanasia, rest upon the notion of freeing us from disability. Such justifications fail to acknowledge the social nature of much suffering and disadvantage and fail to ask who is really suffering? My friend, John, diagnosed as having severe intellectual disability, is one of the happiest and most loving persons I know. I never fail to learn and gain something from my relationship with him, but so often he is seen by others without disability as "suffering." He "must be," after all his very existence challenges the narrow norms dear to those who know that their lives are normal, nice, and successful.

Valuing Disability Knowledge

As I read Hauerwas' critique of Fletcher and reflected on why I had become involved in ethics, I couldn't help feeling that there is something missing. No matter how excellent his analysis and how well he shows the social nature of disability labels such as "retardation," I still left feeling that we need an account of medical ethics, and indeed bioethics in general, which moves beyond talking *about* those with disability to talking *with* those of us with disability. We need accounts of medical ethics which are informed by and commence with the narratives of people with disabilities, and which reflect an ethics which sees the life experience of living with disability as enormously valuable as opposed to inherently negative. We need a bioethics which is able to use the critical insights of disability studies to reflect upon dominant power relations and constructions of knowledge, especially in terms of the dominant discourse of disability which uncritically tend to be used in the practice of medicine and social policy making (see for example Fulcher, 1989).

Those of us who live with disability need the insights of the ethical and theological analysis offered by Stanley Hauerwas. However, his work needs our unmediated insights. We need an ethical approach which writes in conjunction with those with disability and uses the voices and life experience of those with disability as key informants.

That life experience in conjunction with the analysis of Hauerwas can but make the point more successfully. What we require is the beginning of a constructive, critical dialogue between academic medical ethics and people with disabilities. Stanley Hauerwas has deep insights with regard to the nature of suffering, showing significant postmodern insights without the alienating jargon and even idealism which these days accompanies the rhetoric around this area. For example, within the social model's account of disability there is often a failure to recognize that physical conditions such as chronic illness can be more than constructs. While some accounts by people with disabilities have tended to dismiss any notion of disability involving suffering, at the end of the day we need to see that disability is a complex space; more than either a solely medical phenomenon or at the other extreme a mere social construct. As I joked recently from an ICU bed with a colleague: "Of course, this is all a social construct!" I have a variety of experiences of disability. Some of these involve chronic pain, breathlessness, and suffering. For example, the late Bill Williams attests to his situation involving suffering. His journey inherently involves this, and as he shares this with us, we reflect not just on the complexity of disability, but the way in which the suffering and brokenness rejected by the world are crucial components to our human formation (Williams, 1998 a and b).

It is here worth noting that many people with disabilities have tended to reject both theology and ethics as being ableist and irrelevant. The consignment of those of us with disability to marginal placements in medical ethics and its conferences (Clapton, 2000) and the perpetuation of a mainstream theology which largely ignores the insights of theologians with disability, means that we face significant challenges in developing the partnerships between scholars such as Hauerwas and people with disabilities.

The Challenge for Medical Ethics

The practice of medicine today faces increasing challenges. Disability figures as a crucial focal point in the ethical issues confronting not just health care but society in general. The exploration of disability as a social phenomenon in those expanding areas of practice, from genetics to euthanasia, helps us to understand the problem as retarded accounts of ethics rather than retarded individuals. It is those largely taken for granted notions of retardation, disability, suffering, and humanness which need to be critically confronted. The work of Stanley Hauerwas assists us to do this.

Yet, in a world which increasingly questions their validity and existence perhaps the most valuable contribution that people regarded as being retarded have to offer is their very existence. That gift of relationship will help to create a lived, embodied ethics which understands disability as a normal part of life as opposed to something requiring an automatic technological fix. As Hauerwas shows us, the situation of those like my unwitting volunteer student, or my friend John dismissed as retarded, provide the litmus test with regard to our lived ethics. Their situation shows the true nature of what is often claimed as a civil society–a concept which increasingly often does not have a disabled face despite affirmation of diversity in pc circles.

Accordingly, Stanley Hauerwas' work points us to the next important step for medical ethics: moving from talking *about*, to talking and being *in relationship* with, people with disability. The political challenge is whether we truly have the will to do so? The theological challenge asks whether we will embrace the insights from such relationship in theory and practice. Perhaps, in this way we can also start to see our ethics not just in our words but in our actions. I am indebted to Professor Hauerwas for assisting us to think critically about those actions, problematizing the very notions of ethics, therapy, suffering, and retardation which daily oppress people with disability across the globe.

REFERENCES

Clapton, J. (2000). 'Irrelevance Personified: An Encounter Between Bioethics and Disability.' *Interaction*, Vol. 13, No. 3, 2000, pp. 11-15.

Davis, A. (1989). *From Where I Sit*. London: Triangle.

Fulcher, G. (1989). *Disabling Policies?* London: Falmer Press.

Kuhse, H., & Singer, P. (1985). *Should the Baby Live? The Problem of Handicapped Infants*. Oxford: Oxford University Press.

Oliver, M. (1996). *Understanding Disability From Theory to Practice*. Houndmills: MacMillan Press.

Singer, P. (1995). 'Killing Babies isn't always wrong.' *The Spectator*. (16 September) pp. 20-22.

Singer, P., Kuhse, H., Buckle, S., Dawson, K., & Kasimba, P., Eds. (1990), *Embryo Experimentation*. Cambridge: Cambridge University Press.

Williams, W. (1998a). *Naked Before God: The Return of a Broken Disciple*. Harrisburg, PA: Morehouse Publishing.

_____(1998b). *Manna in the Wilderness: A Harvest of Hope*. Harrisburg, PA: Morehouse Publishing.

Chapter 9

Having and Learning to Care
for Retarded Children

Stanley Hauerwas, PhD

(From *Truthfulness and Tragedy: Further investigations into Christian Ethics* (1977, pp. 147-156) Reprinted with permission.

SUMMARY. Hauerwas explores the nature of care. Exploring the notion of parenthood and the purpose of having children, he provides a theological framework which reframes our understanding of all children, including those whom we have chosen to label "mentally retarded."

KEYWORDS. Care, children, mental retardation, theology, community

[Haworth co-indexing entry note]: "Having and Learning to Care for Retarded Children." Hauerwas, Stanley. Co-published simultaneously in *Journal of Religion, Disability & Health* (The Haworth Pastoral Press, an imprint of The Haworth Press, Inc.) Vol. 8, No. 3/4, 2004, pp. 149-159; and: *Critical Reflections on Stanley Hauerwas' Theology of Disability: Disabling Society, Enabling Theology* (ed: John Swinton) The Haworth Pastoral Press, an imprint of The Haworth Press, Inc., 2004, pp. 149-159. Single or multiple copies of this article are available for a fee from The Haworth Document Delivery Service [1-800-HAWORTH, 9:00 a.m. - 5:00 p.m. (EST). E-mail address: docdelivery@haworthpress.com].

A recent letter to the "Wise Man's Corner" of the *St. Anthony Messenger* asked a question I suspect we have all asked, but suppressed for fear of the answer that we might give to it. It read "How does one believe in God, who is supposedly good, when there is so much unhappiness in the world? I have a mentally retarded sister who is in a state institution. On every visiting day it tears me apart to see such ugliness. I know I will never understand God's purpose in allowing these poor human beings to exist with the resulting heartbreak it causes their families every day of their lives. I do very much want to believe in God, but I guess my sister's existence has caused me to resent him. How do I believe?" (*St. Anthony Messenger* 1975, p. 4).

There is much that is theologically naive about this letter. For example, it mistakenly assumes that God is to be held directly responsible for every unfortunate event that occurs in the world. But this kind of theological point fails to come to grips with the agony that gives birth to such letters. For we want to know why or how it is that we can learn to welcome retarded children into our lives without self-pity or false courage. The "Wise Man" attempted to answer this letter by suggesting that the writer contemplate Job and consider the many accounts of people who have had retarded children and the richness they often add to family life.

Yet, while no one can deny that many families have come to see retarded children as a blessing, this response fails to be sufficient. For every case that one can quote that has been morally and spiritually rewarding, another can be found that has been destructive for all the participants. In other words, I am suggesting that our attitudes about retarded children cannot be based on whether or not they enliven certain families. Rather, we must ask what kind of families and communities should we be so we could welcome retarded children into our midst regardless of the happy or unhappy consequences they may bring.

Of course, some may feel to even raise the question of why and how we should learn to accept retarded children is morally and practically a bad faith question. For morally it seems to be prejudicial against those who have made tremendous sacrifices in order to raise and care for retarded children. In other words, it seems to make a matter of doubt out of what they have taken to be a matter of moral necessity. Thus even to raise the question is to change the moral parameters of the case for them.

However, as I hope to show, unless we can give an answer to the question of why such children are to be welcomed into the world we will have no satisfactory moral stance that can give our care of such children moral direction. For as those who work with the retarded soon discover, caring for such children means more than simply providing them with the latest means of therapy or subjecting them to the current forms of educational or behavior-modification theory. For care is not simply "doing" things for these children, even when such "doing" involves our best technologies, but it means knowing how to be with and regard these children with the respect they demand. Thus forms of care with which we approach these children must be guided by our basic beliefs about why we have them at all.

Practically, the question of why we have these children may seem to be nonsense because it is obvious that we cannot avoid them. But in fact this is no longer true. For techniques have been developed, e.g., amniocentesis, that will allow for the early diagnosis and abortion of many children who are suffering from various forms of retardation. Moreover, we are increasingly confronting cases today where parents are refusing life-saving surgery because the child also happens to have been born retarded. Or less dramatically, we know we have often avoided the reality of these children by unnecessary institutionalization.

It, of course, may be thought that these developments are not particularly important for Christians because our attitudes toward abortion preclude the use of amneocentesis for such purposes. Yet I want us to bracket these kinds of concerns about abortion, for I think we will learn more about ourselves, and in particular why abortion is abhorrent to Christians, if we do. For I want to try to show that even if abortion were permissible for Christians we would still have no special or overriding reason to abort a child simply because he or she is destined to be born retarded.

This is the case because the reasons we have these children give essential clues to why we have any children. Moreover, I shall try to suggest that the presence of these retarded children provides us with important skills for how we should learn to care for and raise children not retarded. For contrary to our normal assumptions, the having of children is not a natural event, but rather one of the most highly charged moral events of our lives. The difficulty many feel at the prospect of raising a retarded child is but an indication that we have lost the substantive stories that should inform and give direction to why we have children at all. It is my purpose, therefore, to try to remind us what it is we do when we have children and why the presence of retarded children is so important for helping us understand that story.

CHOOSING OUR CHILDREN

It is a common presumption that we choose or do not choose to have children. Not only do we choose to have children, but since having children has been freed from the necessity of the past, we feel we *should* make having or not having children a matter of choice. Even Catholics who refuse to use contraception still feel that they must describe having children as something they choose to do. For we are people who feel it is important that we have control of our lives, that we not be subject to fate, and one of the ways that we have such control is by choosing to have or not to have children.

Moreover, this seems to be in accordance with our basic responsibilities as parents, for biology does not make us parents. Rather parenting is a role that requires that we be concerned about the conditions into which our children are born and the kind of moral and material care that we can provide them with. Thus the church talks about the importance of "responsible parenthood" indicating that the mere production of children is not a good in itself, but that we should have children in a context that they can receive appropriate forms of care.

Yet it is unclear "how responsible" we must be before we can choose to have children. Does it mean that we must own a good house, have a secure job, and be able to send our children to college? Moreover, what moral prerequisites are required for the having of children, and are moral conditions more important than material conditions? The phrase "responsible parenthood" does little to help us negotiate these kinds of questions.

The ambiguity surrounding these questions has placed a heavy burden on parenting today. For the strong assumption that we choose our children has made us claim unwarranted responsibility for their well-being. Some even go so far as to blame themselves when their children do not get the proper genes to prevent certain aesthetic problems (baldness); or some worry about when their children should be conceived in order that their children are formed by the "best" sperm and ova. Mothers worry if they are giving their children just the right amount of love or attention. This kind of list cataloguing the extraordinary commitments that some parents are willing to accept in order to justify the choice of having children can be extended almost indefinitely. For when there is no reason to have children beyond our individual choice then it seems that we must claim full responsibility or none at all. Against such a background it is clear why more and more people are deciding that they would rather not have children–it is too great a moral burden.

Even though we think we have and should exercise the physical and moral freedom to have children we have no reason, no story, which says why we should exercise this freedom to decide to have children. We thus have children because they are "fun" or because we want to continue the family name; or because our parents or society expect us to have children; or because it just seems to be something that people ought to do. But none of these, or other reasons that are often given for having children, are sufficient to provide us adequate skills for knowing what we should do with children once we have had them. We thus seem trapped to live and raise our children as if the only object is to secure for them a better basis for the acquisition of goods than we had, e.g., that they can go to a better college than we did, have a better job, home, boat, etc. In such a context, however, children end by hating the sacrifices parents have made for their welfare since they perceive the goal was not worth the sacrifice.

For the sacrifice, what we do for our children becomes a way of claiming our children as our own. They are made our property by our choice to have them and by what we do for them–they are our product. As our product, they have no independent existence except as they are able to wrench it from us through psychological and finally physical power.

But ironically, just to the extent that we must choose our children we feel that we must also place a demand on them, namely, that they be perfect. They must be physically and psychologically perfect in order for us to justify all the energy, all the sacrifices that have gone to our choice to have and raise children. After all, who wants to go to all the trouble that children represent for an inferior product. Moreover, it is the sense that children are our total responsibility that makes some parents feel so defeated when their children do something wrong. For if the children are ours, then the natural question when they do something wrong is "Where did we go wrong?" But it is important to notice that such a question, though appearing to be a willingness to assume guilt, is an extraordinary assertion of parental power over the lives of our children. For there is no better way to control others than to claim responsibility for them.

Now I think it is exactly the notion that we choose our children, and the demand that they be perfect, that has created the difficulty of explaining why we have retarded children and moreover corrupted our child-rearing practices for normal children. I want to suggest that it is an extremely odd idea that we *choose* our children. In fact, from our having and rearing children, we know we do not so much choose them, as we discover them as gifts that are not of our making. Indeed, the notion of choosing our children is as misleading as the assumption that we decide to get married (c.f. Hauerwas 1977, pp. 111-119).

Thus I will try to show that if the language of choice is to be used at all in describing our willingness to have children it must be qualified and controlled by the more fundamental metaphor of gift. For only when we understand that our children are gifts can we have an intelligible story that makes clear our duties to them and the form of our care, and in particular the care of our children born retarded, should take.

The Christian Obligation to Have Children

As Christians we do not choose to have our children because we cannot avoid them. This was true before and after contraception became a widespread practice. Rather, Christians (and Jews) have children because it is their duty–they are commanded to do so.

Many may find this terrible, as it seems to rob us of our freedom to decide to have or not to have children. But such a criticism misses the point of why we are obligated to have children, namely, that we are called into the world by a gracious God. For our having children draws on our deepest convictions that God is the Lord of this world, that in spite of all the evidence of misery in this world, it is a world and existence that we can affirm as good as long as we have the assurance that he is its creator and redeemer. That even though we know that this is an existence racked with sin and disobedience, our Lord has provided us with the skills to deal with sin, in ourselves and others, in a manner that will not destroy us or them. Children are thus our promissory note, our sign to present and future generations, that we Christians trust the Lord who has called us together to be his people. (This is the basis of our conviction about abortion, not that life is sacred, but that children should be regarded this way.)

The having of children is hard to make intelligible unless we are members of a people (Hauerwas 1977 b). But we are not just any people: We are a people who are charged to carry the story of God who gives us the basis for our existence as his people. Thus, we do not have our children because we have some obligation to keep the species in tact; or because we wish to furnish our country with a population: population large enough to secure worldly power, but because we are pledged to exist as a Christian community.

The character of that community is therefore crucial for why and how we learn to rear our children. The Christian community is formed by the conviction that the power of this world is not the determining sway of our existence, but rather it is the power we find in the cross of Jesus Christ. Thus, our willingness to have children, our obligation to have children, is one of the ways we serve this community formed by the cross even though the world wishes to deny that a people can exist without the power protected and acquired through the sword.

To many, such a stance will appear foolish or perhaps even immoral. For there is much that could be done that might be considered more important than having children. Children take time and energy, psychologically and physically, that prevents us from being better scholars, important businessmen, serving the poor, or attacking the structures of injustice. But it is the Christian's claim that God's kingdom is not to be built by us that gives us the patience in a world of injustice, to insist that nothing is more important than having and rearing children. We do this not because we assume our children will somehow be better than we are, but because we hope our children will choose to be the next generation of those that carry the story of God in the world. We must remember that our hope is not in our children but in the God who gives us and them grounds of hope.

Of course, this does not mean that everyone who identifies with the Christian faith is called to have children or that each of us should have as many children as we can. Rather, it is to remind us that having children for Christians is a vocation–it is one of the highest callings that we can have in such a community. Some among us (and not just women) will see it as their special vocation to gain the particular skills of learning how to care for and educate children. But all of us who find ourselves members of this people called Christians recognize that this vocation is basic for however we view our own particular calling.

Moreover, this makes clear that as parents we act on the behest of our community as we raise our children. In other words, we do not raise our children to conform just to what we, the child's particular parents, think right. Rather, parents are agents of communities' commitments that both child and parents are or should be loyal to. Indeed, such commitments are the necessary condition to give the child independence from the parents, for the child as well as the parents can appeal to the community for the limits of one another's responsibilities.

That is one of the reasons that the church becomes so important if families are not to he left to their own devices. For unless the child has a community that also provides him or her with symbols of significance beyond the family, then in fact the child is at the mercy of his parents. The church, by insisting that the child is not just the parents' but that the parents have authority insofar as they are agents of the community's values, gives the necessary moral and physical space for children to gain independence from their parents.

Once having children is put in the context of this story and the people formed by it we can see how inappropriate the language of choice is to describe our parenting. For children are not beings created by our wills–we do not choose them–but rather they are called into the world as beings separate and independent from us. They are not ours for they, like each of us, have a Father who wills them as his own prior to our choice of them.

Thus, children must be seen as a gift, for they are possible exactly because we do not determine their right to exist or not to exist. Now it is important to notice that the language of gift involves an extremely interesting grammar. For gifts come to us as a given they are not under our control. Moreover, they are not always what we want or expect and thus they necessarily have an independence from us.

Insofar as gifts are independent they do not always bring joy and surprise, but they equally may bring pain and suffering. But just such pain and suffering is the condition for their being genuine gifts, for gifts that are genuine do not just supply needs or wants, as they would then be subject to our limitations. Rather genuine gifts create needs, that is, they teach us what wants we should have as they must remind us how limited we were without them.

Now children are basic and perhaps the most essential gifts we have because they teach us how to be. That is, they create in us the proper need to want to love and regard another. For love born of need is always manipulative love unless it is based on the regard of the other as an entity that is not in my control but who is all the more valuable because I do not control him. Children are gifts exactly because they draw our love to them while refusing to be as we wish them to be.

But just to the extent that we realize that our children are a duty can we also be freed from the excessive concern and claims of responsibility associated with our decision to have children. For contrary to contemporary assumptions duties bring freedom by helping us learn to accept the proper moral limitations of being human. We destroy ourselves and our children just to the extent that we act as if there are no such limits.

The Retarded as Gifts

Thus we must learn to accept the retarded into our lives as a peculiar and intense form of how we should regard all children. They are not, to be sure, the kind of children we would choose to have, for we would wish on no one any unnecessary suffering or pain. But they are not different from other children insofar as any child is not of our choosing.

Children, Suffering, and the Skill to Care

It is of course true that retarded children destroy our plans and fantasies about what we wish our children to be. They thus call us to reality quicker than most children, as they remind us that the plans we have for our children may not be commensurate with the purpose for which we have children at all. Thus, these retarded children are particularly special gifts to remind us that we have children not that they be a success, not for what they may be able to do for the good and betterment of mankind, but because we are members of a people who are gathered around the table of Christ.

I want to be very clear about this. I am not suggesting that Christians should rejoice that their children are born retarded rather than normal. Rather, I am suggesting that as Christians the story that informs and directs why we have children at all provides us with the skill to know how to welcome these particular children into our existence without telling ourselves self-deceiving stories about our heroism for doing so. For such heroic stories can also serve to subject the retarded child to forms of care that they should not be forced to undergo.

For example, such heroic stories can lead us to forms of sentimental care and protection that rob these children of the demands to grow as they are able. For the love of the retarded, like any love, must be hard if we are to not stifle the other in overprotective care. Or to, care for these children as if they are somehow specially innocent–that is "children of God"–is to rob them of the right to be the kind of selfish, grasping, and manipulative children other children have the right to be. Retarded children are not to be cared for because they are especially loving, though some of them may be, but because they are children. We forget that there is no more disparaging way to treat another than to assume that they can do nothing wrong.

But just as the retarded child is a gift like any other child, they also require special skills if we are to care for them appropriately. What is important is not that we Christians have retarded children, but that we know why and to what end we have them. To have them in order to witness to what nice people we are is only another subtle way to use them. We have them because they are children–no special reason beyond that needs to be given–but as children they present special needs that we must know how to meet responsibly. For we must know how to care for them in ways that respect their independence from us as their existence as well as our own, it is grounded in the fact that we are each called to service in God's kingdom.

The Care of the Retarded

How one cares for the retarded child will of course differ in terms of the kind of retardation and from child to child–no two Downs syndrome children, just like no two normal children, are the same. Moreover, I have no competency to try to suggest what kind of care or training is better than another. However, I think it is important and necessary to try to articulate some general guidelines that should govern our care of retarded children irrespective of the kind of retardation and the techniques best to deal with it.

For the great temptation in caring for the retarded, as with any child, is to make them conform to what we think they should want to be, namely, "normal. " We thus often care for the retarded on the assumption that our task is to make them as much like the rest of us as we can. But as I have suggested, the very way we learn to accept these children into our lives requires us to learn to see and love them as gifts which are not at our disposal.

We must, therefore, be very careful we do not impose on them a form of life that is given birth by our frustration that they are not and cannot be like us. For example, the so-called "principle of normalization" is a valuable check against the sentimental and often cruel care of the retarded that tries to spare them the pain of learning basic skills of living. But as an ideology it tends to suggest that our aim is to make the retarded "normal." This, of course, ignores entirely that we have no clear idea of what it means to be "normal." Thus, in the name of name of "normalcy" we stand the risk of making the retarded conform to convention because they lack the power to resist.

As Milton Mayeroff reminds us, to care for another person, in the most significant sense, is to help him grow and actualize himself (Mayeroff 1971, p. 1). That is, to care for others is to help them establish an independent existence from us-not to be under our power. "To help another person grow is at least to help him to care for something or someone apart from himself, and it involves encouraging and assisting him to find and create areas of his own in which he is able to care. Also, it is to help that other person to come to care for himself, and by becoming responsive to his own need to care to become responsible for his own life" (Mayeroff 1971, pp. 10-11). The retarded must be cared for in a way, therefore, that they are seen to have the ability to care for others as we care for them.

To care requires the supporting virtues of patience–for we must learn to wait even when the other fails; honesty–for we must learn how to tell the truth to the other even when it is unpleasant; trust–to let the other take the risk of the unknown; and humor–that the other knows that no mistake is a decisive defeat. Therefore, the kind of care required for learning to live with the retarded requires a substantive story that will give us the patience, honesty, trust, and humor to provide them with the space to acquire such virtues of care themselves.

Such virtues and story are required for all child-rearing, but it may be that they are especially intensified in learning how to care for the retarded. For to know how to care for the retarded requires the special skill not to be over-protective. Such a skill is possible when we have the confidence that the destiny of retarded children is not finally in our hands–that they and we are both sustained by a power beyond our capacity. In the presence of such a power we have the grounds for taking the risk of caring for the retarded exactly because their existence and ours are called forth by the God we have come to know in the history of Israel and the cross of Christ. For we have learned that this power refused to sustain our existence as if our existence is an end in itself. Rather, we are sustained by service to God who asks nothing more from us than to be his people who continue to have time in the business of this world to have children, even if they are retarded.

REFERENCES

Hauerwas. Stanley. (1977a). 'Rights, duties, and experimentation in children.' In *Appendix to Report and Recommendations on Research Involving Children of the National Commission for the Protection of Human Subjects*. DHEW Publication No. (OS) 77-0005.

Hauerwas, Stanley. (1977b). 'The Family: Theological and Ethical Reflections.' In Van Kussrow and Richard Baepler (Eds.) (1977), *Changing American Life Styles*. Valparaiso: University of Valparaiso Press. pp. 11-119.

Mayerhoff, Milton. (1971). *On Caring*. New York: Harper & Rowe.

Chapter 10

The Retarded, Society, and the Family: The Dilemma of Care

Stanley Hauerwas, PhD

[Hauerwas, Stanley. (1986) *The Retarded, Society, and the Family,* in *Suffering Presence: Theological Reflections on Medicine, the Mentally Handicapped, and the Church.* London: Continuum International Publishing, pp 189–210.] Reprinted with permission.

SUMMARY. This paper develops the theme of care which was begun in chapter 9. Here Hauerwas focuses on the importance of the family in the process of caring for people with developmental disabilities. He explores the motivation behind parenting and offers some piercing insights into *why* we have children and the ways in which our motivation for having children impacts upon the experience of having a child with a developmental disability.

The author would like to thank Anne Hauerwas and Mark Sherwindt for their criticism of an earlier version of this paper.

[Haworth co-indexing entry note]: "The Retarded, Society, and the Family: The Dilemma of Care." Hauerwas, Stanley. Co-published simultaneously in *Journal of Religion, Disability & Health* (The Haworth Pastoral Press, an imprint of The Haworth Press, Inc.) Vol. 8, No. 3/4, 2004, pp. 161-179; and: *Critical Reflections on Stanley Hauerwas' Theology of Disability: Disabling Society, Enabling Theology* (ed: John Swinton) The Haworth Pastoral Press, an imprint of The Haworth Press, Inc., 2004, pp. 161-179. Single or multiple copies of this article are available for a fee from The Haworth Document Delivery Service [1-800-HAWORTH, 9:00 a.m. - 5:00 p.m. (EST). E-mail address: docdelivery@haworthpress.com].

KEYWORDS. Care, families, disability, theology

THE RETARDED AND THE FAMILY:
OUR UNEXAMINED ASSUMPTIONS

It is a commonplace that the family, in particular the family of retarded children, should have the primary responsibility for the care of their children. This is not simply because parents, due to their proximity, are assumed to know best what their children need. Rather, our society's commitment to care physically and morally for children through the agency of their parents is based on the profound assumption that the family has or should have moral priority over all other institutions and values. Thus, Gliedman and Roth, in their book *The Unexpected Minority*, argue that the parent's rights over the child take precedence over the professional's personal moral views. To put it bluntly, the professional exists to further the parent's vision of the handicapped child's future. Should the professional disagree, he has every right to try to *persuade* the parent to adopt a different view. He also has every right to give advice when the parent is confused and seeks guidance and emotional support. But except in the most extreme instances of parental incompetence and brutality, such as child abuse, the professional has no right to use his immense moral and practical power to intimidate or to manipulate the parent (Gliedman and Roth, p. 1979, p. 104).

The fact that parents are often manipulated, if not bullied, by professionals does not mean that the primacy of the family is not a working norm for our society. Indeed, we can and do criticize the tendency toward professional dominance exactly because of our deep and profound adherence to the family as the locus of moral and physical support for children. Parents have the right to make decisions that will affect their children's lives because we assume that parents are, or should be, the best representatives of their children's interest.

However, like most commonplaces, our assumption about our commitment to the family is seldom made explicit, much less subjected to rigorous analysis. Why do we think the family should have such high moral status or why should parents make the basic decisions concerning the care of their children? For example, why do we support the presumption that simply because a man and a woman are able to conceive a child they should be the ones to raise and determine what should or should not be done for that child? Biological identity certainly is not sufficient to make one a parent, for we view "being a parent" as fundamentally a moral role with definite tasks and privileges.

Exactly what that moral competency involves is not a matter we subject to rigorous investigation; rather, we tend to assume that if a couple is capable of producing a child they probably also have the "maturity" to know how to care for and raise children. We assume this even though we are increasingly aware that this is simply not the case. The problem of teenage pregnancy is but the tip of the iceberg, as many people who have children lack any sense whatsoever of the moral skills required for becoming a parent.

It is important to note that the question is not whether parents have the material resources necessary to have children, but whether they have the moral resources for such a task. For the priority of the family for the care and nurture of children is primarily a moral commitment that need not, though it often does, imply the presence of economic means to provide that care. We might well think some families, such as those who have retarded children, should receive material support from elsewhere without qualifying our assumption that the family is morally primary. However, in our kind of society, it is hard to maintain the independence of such a moral commitment where equal financial independence is lacking. The rule still pertains that where the queen's shilling appears, the queen is not far behind.

The fact that we do not subject to rigorous analysis our assumption of the primacy of the family for the care of children is not simply due to intellectual obstinacy. Rather, our willingness to allow anyone capable of conceiving children to do so is based on our profound commitment to individual freedom. In the name of individual rights, we refrain as a society from interfering with a couple's decision to have children, no matter how incompetent we think they might be. Moreover, we also refrain from trying to determine, once children are present, how parents should care for their children in the name of protecting the "sacredness" of the family.

In the process, we fail to notice that the appeal to "freedom" or "rights" of people to be parents distorts the traditional basis for the moral primacy of the family. Traditionally, parents were assumed to have overriding responsibility for their children because they were assumed capable and could be held accountable for performing certain duties. For example, the family was granted priority to the state in matters dealing with education of children because it was assumed that the family had the responsibility to transmit the wisdom of our culture. Presently, however, appeals to these substantive responsibilities seem to qualify the freedom of the individual, especially if they are in any way used to set social policy involving the having and raising of children. We think we have a right to become a parent irrespective of the kind of person and thus parent we may be or become.

Moreover, I suspect most of us feel no great need to analyse or make explicit the moral presumptions surrounding parenthood, because we think we know what we are doing when we become parents. We have children because we assume that it will he a rewarding experience both for them and for us. We look forward to having children, assuming that the business of raising children is a normal task that requires no extraordinary moral or intellectual skills. Almost anyone can do it, though there may be a few rocky moments for even the best prepared.

I suspect that one of the reasons the discovery that our child is retarded comes as such a shock and jolt is that our assumptions about why we have children have seemed too obvious to examine. After all, this is not what we counted on and certainly does not seem part of the implicit agreement that we assumed we were making in our decision to have a child. We were willing to devote large resources of time, energy, and money for the rearing of this child on the assumption that we would be dealing with a fairly normal being. To have to raise and care for a retarded child simply seems unfair, given our assumptions about having a child in the first place. All those plans for camping trips, football games, or intellectual sharing of ideas too quickly die in the struggle to attain the minimal skills. Suddenly, rather than learning to read by three, we are rejoicing at learning bladder control by twelve.

That such is the case I think also accounts for the reaction of parents of normal children to parents of retarded children. The former do not like to get too close to the latter, since their very presence is a reminder that none of us are very sure what we are doing when we become parents. Parents of retarded children soon discover that most of their relations with other adults, outside the work place, involve those who also have retarded children. Parents of retarded children are often regarded with a great deal of suspicion by parents of normal children as the latter suspect that the extraordinary time and energy put into caring for these children–time that rarely seems worth it, given the level of accomplishment–is really but a way of tying to assuage guilt for having had the bad luck of having a retarded child in the first place.

We thus prefer to keep the retarded and their parents at arm's length, because their presence raises a question most of us prefer remain unasked–namely, what commitments are involved in being a parent that seems to require we care for these children? We assume that our commitment to the family as the locus of care for children is sufficient to answer this question; however, I have tried to suggest that our inability to spell out what is involved morally in being a parent makes that an extremely ambiguous undertaking. I will try to show that it is not enough to assume parents ought to care for their children, retarded and non-retarded, for that assumption simply is not sufficient to inform us about what kind of care parents should provide. Unless we know more about the latter than the former, commitment loses its moral intelligibility. Indeed, unless these additional aspects of the moral claims implicated in parenting are made explicit, appeals to the priority of the family for the care of children can have the ironic effect of leaving us morally groundless and defenseless when the care provided for the child is literally destructive.

The Priority of the Family:
The Example of Parents of the Retarded

I am not going to try to provide a theory for why we think the family should have priority in caring for children. Nor am I going to appeal to any abstract principles to try to suggest the kind of responsibilities that we have as parents for our children. What we must admit is that our culture simply lacks any consensus sufficient to provide a satisfactory response to either of these questions (Hauerwas 1981). Rather, I want to draw our attention to what parents of retarded children do, even if they often are unable to say why it is they do what they do. For it is my contention that they have more to teach us than anyone about why we are right in thinking that the family is and should be the primary locus for care of children, both normal and retarded.

I think this way of proceeding is partly justified by the obvious fact that most of us learn what it means to be a parent from our children. Their needs teach us our responsibilities. We simply learn to be a parent through the thousands of small things that we learn to do on a day-to-day basis to meet the demands of sustaining and raising our children. What we must learn to do is to say what it is that we have learned. Indeed, one of the primary reasons inhibiting many from becoming parents today involves our inability to pass the skills of parenting from one generation to another. For parenting is not a "natural" role, but involves skills that can be acquired only by learning them from others. Unfortunately, we seem to lack people who have confidence that they possess those skills to the degree that they are capable of handing them on to us and teaching them to others.

The only justification for looking at parents of retarded children is that they are taught their responsibilities more quickly and more intensely than most of us. They learn from the beginning that our children have a claim on us even though they do not turn out to be what we expected. Normal children, of course, also always turn out to be quite different than we expected, but we are not made so intensely aware of the implications of that fact in those cases.

Parents of retarded or multiple-handicapped children learn from the beginning they must fight for their children. In this regard it is illuminating to listen to Helen Brown's account of a time soon after the birth of her multiple-handicapped daughter, an account that I suspect could be duplicated by countless other parents of retarded children. "At home we couldn't discuss Karen. Richard seemed brave and strong. Unknown to me, he and my mother visited Karen at the hospital almost every day. But between us, there was only grief-stricken silence. No one wanted to talk about Karen, no one offered comfort and advice. The specialists were aloof and matter-of-fact. My mother and husband were as overcome as I was. My neighbors–most of them pregnant or new mothers themselves–only brought home to me my loss. I turned at last to the doctor who had delivered Karen and who supplied my only comfort.

> 'Have another baby as soon as possible,' he told me.
> 'But maybe, just maybe, Karen will come home, and she'll need me.'
> 'Please listen to the experts,' he said. 'Be brave and strong. You're a perfectly healthy young woman, and there's no reason why you can't have a dozen more children. Let this child go.'

I couldn't give up my desperate hope that she would turn out to be perfect and well. I couldn't make the idea of another baby seem like a reality. Only Karen was real, even though I hadn't seen her since she was born.

> 'You would be ruining your life and your marriage if you tried to bring her home,' the doctor said. 'Right now she needs constant supervision and medication, and if she survives, there's no telling what she'll be like. Put her out of your mind.'
> 'At least let me see her.'
> 'There's nothing you can do for her. You'd only be breaking your heart.'
> 'She must need her mother. Babies need their mothers.'
> 'She doesn't know the difference, believe me. The best thing to do is forget her.'

Wouldn't it have been wonderful–to be able to forget her? If I could have done that, it might have been best, but I was haunted by the memory of her, the child of my dreams, the only two times I had ever seen her: first perfect and beautiful, then red and convulsed, through the window of the hospital nursery. I tried to forget, but I couldn't" (Brown 1976, pp. 33-34).

That such a conversation is not unusual is well-documented in Rosalyn Darling's *Families Against Society* (Darling 1979). Darling began her study to test whether in fact handicapped children have the low self-esteem that most theories of self-esteem seem to suggest they should. She soon discovered that their self-esteem was not significantly different from that of normal control groups. On investigating why this might be the case, she discovered that if parents of handicapped children regard them positively, then their children are likely to have high self-esteem, regardless of the views of anyone else.

That parents of retarded children learn to regard their children with respect, however, is no simple process. Indeed, Darling found that prior to the birth or later discovery of their child's handicap most parents share our society's general negative judgment about such children. As one of Darling's respondents says, "I knew nothing about mental retardation–just the vague stories one hears when growing up. These were 'people to be shunned.' I was ignorant of any factual knowledge" (Darling 1979, p. 124). It is only through intense day-to-day interaction with their children that parents find the means to challenge and change their own stereotypes of what it means to be handicapped as well as find the means to challenge the stereotypes of our society. Darling's book, therefore, is primarily an account of how parents were taught by their handicapped children to be parents.

Most parents of handicapped children, according to Darling, go through a series of stages which she characterizes from anomic to activism. At first, parents are simply shocked into a state of helplessness by the knowledge that something is seriously wrong with their child. Their feeling of helplessness is only exaggerated by professionals who do not tell them what is wrong with their child in the interest of protecting them from the truth. Not only was the anxiety of parents increased by the evasiveness of many of the professionals, but many parents felt that doctors tended to be overly negative about the description of their child's condition. Thus, Darling quotes some parents reporting: "The doctor called me and said that there was a question about the baby's health, that there was concern over whether we had a 'good baby,' and some doctors seem to think he's mongoloid," and even, "The pediatrician said, 'Your baby has_____ Syndrome. Here's some information you can read about it, but don't worry, she probably won't live'" (Darling 1979, p. 133).

Darling characterizes this first stage as anomic to denote the parents 'feelings of helplessness and lack of support in the face of what appears at the time to be an overwhelming tragedy. The temptation of self-pity and a concern for the future quickly become all-consuming for many parents. But interestingly enough this period often tends be short-lived if the parents receive support from the family and friends, and, in particular, if they have interaction with the child. For example, Darling was told:

> I talked to a nurse and then I felt less resentment. I said I was afraid, and she helped me feed the baby. . . . Then my girlfriend came to see me. She had just lost her husband, and we sort of supported each other. . . . By the time she came home, I loved her. When I held her the first time, I felt love and worried if she would live. As time goes on, you fall in love. You think, "this kid's mine and nobody's gonna take her away from me." I think by the time she was two weeks old I wasn't appalled by her anymore. (Darling 1979, p. 136)

After recovering from their initial anomie, Darling suggests parents begin what she calls a "seekership" phase. The greatest need they feel is for information, not just about their child's condition, but about what can be done. Too often friends and relatives at this point try to help by denying the seriousness of the child's condition. Even more troubling is the common complaint of parents that the medical treatment their children received is not only often inadequate but also dehumanizing. Almost all parents of retarded children report that:

> My pediatrician kept after me to put him away [in an institution]. (We finally changed pediatricians.) Our new pediatrician gushed all over us at first. . . . But then, he never touched Billy. I always had to move him for him. We were never left in the waiting room. It was like I was an embarrassment. When Billy was in the hospital our old pediatrician stuck his head in the door and said, "it's too bad he couldn't go [die]. . . . " The doctors on rounds would talk outside our door and they ripped apart parents who keep their [severely handicapped] children. (Darling 1979, p. 151)

Another parent reported that taking your child to the doctor is like "when you take your dog to the vet . . . not many doctors pick him up and try to communicate with him as a child" (Darling 1979, p. 151). That there does exist a wide discrepancy between the attitudes of pediatricians and parents of handicapped children does seem to be the case if Darling's research is anything close to being accurate. Thus, in her interviews with pediatricians, they almost all testified to their dislike of caring for handicapped (and in particular, retarded) children. They usually recommend institutionalization. In the words of one physician, "I have yet to see a mother who has not been adversely affected by having a mongoloid child in the house. Despite the fact that women protest and act in a good, competent way, I really feel that it's affected their lives in a way that robs their being a better person. If one is to think that the object is to make a better life, it interferes with that object. Seeing these people over the years . . . the look in their eyes, their demeanor–it's compensatory, not fulfilling" (Darling 1979, p. 216).

Most parents soon learn not to look for miracles or cures. All they want is to find a competent pediatrician or specialist who will treat their child "like a person." Unfortunately, parents are often forced to spend a great deal of their time simply trying to find a physician who is able to view their child in this manner.

During this period, parents increasingly discover that they do not have great difficulty in learning to accept their children as they learn that they are able to meet their needs. Interestingly enough, this adds to the parents' self-esteem as they realize that they are capable of more than they expected. The difficulty comes not in accepting their own children, but in our society's unwillingness to accept these children as part of our public lives. Parents soon discover that their own matter-of-fact acceptance of their children and their handicaps is not widely shared in our society. They often must learn to deal with the pained embarrassment, if not outright hostility, that results from bringing their children out in public.

Parents learn, however, that public rejection of their children is one of the small obstacles they must encounter. As their children grow older and as their parents seek education, physical, and recreational services, they discover that such services are inadequate or do not exist at all. As one mother put it, they soon realize that "Our society is not geared for the retarded. We used to send them all away and now we don't know what to do with them" (Darling 1979, p. 178). As a result, parents learn it is not enough to try to find the service available for their children. They must learn to fight to establish and create the kind of care their children rightly deserve. Some, Darling denotes, attribute this kind of advocacy for their children to guilt, but she suggests that such "parental behavior is easily understandable within the context of parents trying to 'do their job' as parents in an inhospitable society" (Darling 1979, p. 181).

Thus, parents enter what Darling calls an "advocacy" period as they find they must create institutions and programs to provide better care for their children. They become crusaders willing to challenge the at best sentimental attitude and care offered by our society by demanding their children he treated with respect. It is of interest to note that Darling discovered that often lower-income and less-educated parents become the most effective advocates for their children, as they seem to have had more experience in dealing with unresponsive bureaucracies.

The great strength of parents of retarded children is their lack of illusion about their children. They refuse to let their children be destroyed by sentimental kindness that ends only by reinforcing our stereotypes about what the "retarded are able to do." They demand that our society provide the training that will allow their children to attain the level of activity of which they are capable, even if such training proves painful for their children.

In this respect, the parents of retarded children have often faced the reality of their situation with more insight than most of us assume is the case. For example, all of Darling's respondents suggested they would have preferred that their child not be born with handicaps because they would not wish their child so burdened. Once their children were born, however, they discovered they loved them no less for their handicap and gained new confidence in themselves as they learned to deal with the demands such children placed on them. This confidence, moreover, gave them the strength to take on a much larger struggle against the ways in which our society ignores or flatly rejects the retarded.

The extent of that struggle has recently been depicted by John Gliedman and William Roth in their book *The Unexpected Minority*. They point out that the most decisive disadvantage the handicapped face in our society is not the most overt forms of discrimination that come through our educational and economic structures, which are certainly real enough, but the very categories through which we understand the handicapped. In contrast to most analyses of the handicapped which suggest that the problem is getting better medical and social help for the handicapped, Gliedman and Roth argue that the handicapped should be understood as an oppressed minority group.

It is not that Gliedman and Roth are opposed to the handicapped getting better medical and educational help, but what is crucial is the presupposition on which that help is determined. For example, they suggest that they began their study believing "that the traditional definition of the handicapped child's needs was perfectly satisfactory—that all that was really required was more of the same kind of services for handicapped children. Only gradually did we come to see our initial error. By failing to think through the implications of the 'civil rights lens' for the child, we had unwittingly committed ourselves to making the same kinds of mistakes about disability that were made about other groups of disadvantaged children a generation ago" (Gliedman and Roth 1979, p. x).

This mistake, according to Gliedman and Roth, consists in the failure to recognize or understand the implications that a "handicap" is fundamentally a social construction. As a society we tend to diagnose handicaps as disease-like states. This entails, however, a vicious circle. "Our misconceptions about the incapacitating consequences of a disability cause us to see the person as a deviant, as one who cannot fit into any of the roles assumed by normals in everyday life. Then the culturally determined associations of deviance with disease states encourage us to single out those aspects of the individual that are disease like. By assigning a medical cause to the paraplegic's deviance—his putative inability to assume any normal role in society—lay society denies its responsibility for excluding the individual from normal life" (Gliedman and Roth 1979, p. 11). What we must come to understand, they argue, is that our apparent "objective" perceptions of handicaps as socially incapacitating biological conditions are perceptual products of a prior, and often unconscious, social construction (Gliedman and Roth 1979, p. 15).

Gliedman and Roth note that on the surface this way of identifying the handicapped seems just and fair. After all, to be handicapped is not viewed as punishment (at least not overtly). Nor is it invested with mysterious supernatural associations. Rather, we assume that we are taking a scientific approach—that since the handicapped are portrayed as the victims of impersonal accidents, disease processes, and genetic imperfections, stigma, and prejudice are out of place. The handicapped are excused because they cannot help being handicapped any more than someone can help being sick. Therefore, what is called for is understanding and assistance (Gliedman and Roth 1979, p. 20).

What we fail to see, however, is that by interpreting handicaps in terms of the medical model, we have in effect robbed the handicapped of what they need most. The medical model obscures the essential fact about the handicapped person's situation, namely, that the disadvantages that result from most handicaps derive more from our society's prejudices than from the handicap itself. The medical model is particularly destructive for the handicapped in that it puts them in a disastrous psychological and sociological situation: They must define themselves as permanently dependent if they are to receive the advantages of the sick role. Moreover, this robs handicapped persons of their most effective means of doing something about their situation, namely, politics. Because issues of health and disease are matters which are thought dealt with primarily in terms of charity, the handicapped are denied the resource necessary to understand or deal with the discrimination they experience for what it is, namely, they have been robbed unjustly of power that is rightfully theirs and which can only be regained politically. The burden of Gliedman and Roth's presentation is to show that once this has happened, the various professions designed to help the handicapped, often with the best will and enthusiasm for the task, are but another form of discrimination as they depoliticize the handicapped person's situation.

Without denying the social nature of any understanding of a "handicap," Gliedman and Roth's point can be misleading if the implication is drawn that all identification of handicaps are arbitrary and discriminating. There is something wrong with someone who is retarded just as there is something wrong with the fact I have flat feet. The retarded have real disabilities and they need aid, and of the best kind, to help them deal with their handicap.

Gliedman and Roth, however, are right that retardation is a social construction in terms of how a handicap is understood and how it is interpret to limit the retarded's activity. Moreover, they are right to suggest that retardation, as a social construction, is particularly destructive for anyone so described as it is assumed to describe a condition that determines a person's every activity. Everything we are and do is done as one who is "retarded." What is needed is discriminating forms of judgement that denote those aspects of life and activities where retardation simply is irrelevant. But that, it seems, is exactly what we do not have, and as a result Gliedman and Roth are right to suggest that retardation too often becomes a self-fulfilling prophecy that unfortunately is perpetuated by the very theories and people who want to "help" the retarded.

Parents and Professionals

As I suggested earlier, Gliedman and Roth think that the only source capable of breaking this vicious cycle is for parents of retarded to reclaim their right to determine the kind of care their children should receive. It is parents, who often have not been schooled on theories about what their retarded children can and cannot do, that are able to demand more from those who would too easily acquiesce to the limitations of the medical model. No one can be around parents of retarded children long, people who, to be sure, have often sought and dealt with one professional after another in the hopes of finding help for their child, without realizing that these are among the few people in our society who have learned to deal with the tyranny of the "expert."

That they have done so is largely because they have learned to trust their own judgment when dealing with their child. To be sure, they are more knowledgeable than most of us and they have learned, often painfully, that experts disagree. However, their fundamental ability to resist the professional comes from their passionate commitment to make the expert see their children as they have learned to see their children, i.e., as fellow members of the human community whose struggle with the limits and possibilities of their existence deserves our most profound respect and support.

I think it would be a mistake, however, to interpret the relationship between the retarded and their parents as only a one-way street. For I have observed that the retarded have often done marvelous things for their parents, not the least of which is their requiring their parents, in their role as advocates, to come in contact with others who are as different from them as their own children. In the process, unlike most of us, their parents have also learned basic political skills for the formation of communities as they learn to work and plan together in order to secure their children a better life.

Even more important to my mind is how parents of retarded children discover what the world is like through their children. The necessity of caring for such children requires us quickly to break through the myths and deceptions that our social order encourages us to accept—one of which is that life is about being a perpetual member of the Pepsi® generation. Our society encourages us to think that we can be a good people without suffering, that we can pursue our own interests with little thought of what it does to others. Parents of children born retarded know better. And because they know better they are able to insist that our society set their children not as permanently ill, but simply as different.

Much more could be said about such matters, but enough has been said to make my basic point, namely, that through their children parents of retarded children are trained to be parents in a manner that illuminates what it means morally to be a parent for anyone. Nothing, I have said, of course, commits me to the thesis that parents of the retarded, any more than the retarded themselves, are free from perverse distortions of their role. Indeed, many people unable to face their retarded children, abandon them literally or at least psychologically. Or there are parents who unduly emphasize and reinforce their child's handicap as a means to enhance their own status. We all to some extent thrive on the need to be needed and it is hard indeed to learn to force independence on those who seem so dependent.

No doubt other equally subtle and more destructive behavior could be depicted involving the way some parents of retarded children manage themselves and their children. That perversions occur does not show that our commitment to the family as the primary locus for care of children is wrong. Rather, the perversions are but indications of the extraordinary demands that such commitments entail. By calling attention to the way parents of retarded children are taught to be parents, I have tried to remind us how certain kinds of responsibilities give substance to our assumption that the family should have primary responsibility for the rearing of and caring for children.

Before I try to make something out of all this, however, let me qualify an impression that I may have created. For the "heavy" in the above account appears to be the professional–the doctor, researcher, social worker, teacher, and many others. To be sure, many professionals surely deserve the criticism as made, but many do not. Many are dedicated people who see retarded people clearly and often more clearly than parents themselves. Indeed, all parents need help from others, whether they be "professionals" or not, to jar them out of too easily accepted assumptions about the limits or possibilities of their children's capabilities.

The problem with making the professional the bad guy, however, involves a more fundamental mistake than simply slandering many of the dedicated and competent professions who deal with the retarded. For when the professional is made the primary object of criticism, we fail to diagnose adequately our situation. The problem and the dilemma is more profound than simply challenging the dominance of the professional. For the truth is that the state and the professional who often acts as the agent of the state, have increasingly been called on to be more directly involved in the care of the retarded because the family has simply abdicated its role. But, as I will try to show, that families have done so is not simply because they are morally deficient, though some may be, but because as a society we lack a consensus that can inform expectations for child care by parents and what kind of appropriate support is should thus be provided by our society and state to support that care.

The Dilemma of Care

Therefore, rather than continuing my paean to parents of the retarded, we need to step back and ask some critical questions about what I have been doing. For, in effect, I have used a persuasive example to do the work of argument and in the process belied the ambiguity of our commitment to care for the retarded by and through the family. I have tried to suggest why we rightly think that the family is and should be the primary locus of care for the retarded by calling attention to how the retarded train their parents to care for them. By appealing to the everyday, but in many ways quite heroic, struggle of parents to secure adequate care for their handicapped children, I have reinforced our assumption that the family should have priority for the care of the retarded.

By proceeding by way of example, however, I have weighed the case in a manner that fails to take adequate account of the dilemma raised by focusing on care of the retarded through the family. Simply put, all I have shown is that our society supports the formal commitment that children should be cared for by their parents, but that society does not and cannot require parents to give the kind of cue that my examples suggest and which most of us find so admirable. In other words, I have reinforced our assumption that the retarded should be cared for through the agency of the family by suggesting, without adequate support, that such care will be of the kind my examples display. I can make this more concrete in terms of some of the agonizing dilemmas that occur in almost any hospital with a neonatal unit. Often children are born who, in addition to being retarded, also have some other accompanying difficulty that requires surgical correction if the child is to live. The most famous case is that of a Down's syndrome child born with duodenal atresia whose parents refused the surgery necessary to stop the child from starving to death. More difficult cases involve questions about how much should be done or how much parents should do to keep alive children suffering from spina bifida. Many assume the parents of the Down's syndrome child were clearly wrong not to secure adequate medical attention for their child, but when confronted by the multiple and severe problems often associated with spina bifada, the case is not so clear and the correct paths not so sure. I am not interested at this point in arguing the case one way or the other; rather, I simply want to point out that if we grant that the family is the primary locus for care of the retarded, this by no means insures that the retarded will receive the kind of care we think they should receive.

A still more troubling issue is raised by programs to prevent retardation. Many are rightly concerned to prevent retardation. No one would wish that a child be born retarded when it can be avoided through proper prenatal care and adequate infant and early childhood maintenance. But the language of prevention when applied to retardation is more ambiguous than is often recognized.

For we can prevent cancer without destroying the subject of cancer. But when we set out to "prevent" retardation, there is no way the disease entity can be separated from the diseased. If we prevent retardation, it means we must be prepared to prevent, if not eliminate, the retarded. Such a project becomes particularly problematic if we take seriously Gieldman and Roth's contention that retardation is as much a social construction as a biological or medical category.

The problem of prevention can be graphically illustrated by asking whether we, as a society, ought to encourage all women thirty-five and older to undergo amniocentesis. By asking this question, I do not mean to weight the question of abortion one way or the other. Rather, I am simply trying to explore what such a suggestion would mean for our attitudes about the retarded and in particular the responsibilities of parents for them.

For example, it is quickly becoming a general assumption that a woman thirty-five or older should have amniocentesis. As a result, anyone who has a retarded child in later life is viewed with a good deal of suspicion, if not outright hostility. After all, they should have known better and taken the appropriate steps. But why do we think that? Why do we assume that it is the task of parents to avoid having children who may be retarded? Or perhaps better, how far do we think that people ought to go in order to avoid having retarded children?

Moreover, our concern with prevention of the retarded may have unanticipated social policy implications. It has been our assumption that a reduction in the number of retarded children will translate into more public dollars for their care. However, this by no means follows, as the diminishing social budget we face over the next few years might well turn in the other direction. The fewer who need to be cared for might mean that our society would find it less costly simply to make parents do the best they can, and if they abdicate this responsibility, the state can warehouse their children more easily. Or still more troubling, as amniocentesis becomes more common, some may think they have little responsibility to support with public money a mistake the parents could have easily avoided.

Perhaps even more troubling are the moral implications of amniocentesis as a public policy. For public policy involves not just issues of distribution but also assumptions about what kind of people we ought to be. Does amniocentesis imply that we should be willing to be parents only if we can assume we are working with a "perfect" child? And if so, how are we to determine what such a child should look like?

By raising these issues I do not *mean* to suggest that amniocentesis should never be used, but I raise the questions about amniocentesis and the other issues only to illustrate my contention that our appeal to the family as the locus for the care of the retarded simply is not sufficient to tell us how the family should care for the retarded. Indeed, as I have tried to suggest, the commitment to the family in itself can as easily result in individual retarded children receiving less than adequate care and may mean that the retarded receive even less support as the object of social policy.

Thus we find ourselves in a dilemma. We are inheritors of a tradition that presumes that the family is our central social institution for the care of children, but we have no idea what the family should be. This dilemma, however, serves to remind us that the family is not an end in itself or an isolatable social entity, but requires moral direction and support from a community. The family does not exist just to exist, but like any other significant institution it needs purposes and tasks. This is exactly what our society is unsure about, since to specify tasks for the family with any kind of moral specificity appears as a threat to our "freedom." As a result, we talk much and loudly about the value of the family in our society, having little idea why it in fact has worth.

In this respect, issues raised by the relation of the family and the retarded are but one aspect of the larger problem of the status of the family in our society. We are often told the family is in crisis, but there is little consensus about the nature of cause of the crisis. Indeed, many deny that there is any crisis at all, calling attention to the fact that the family remains very strong, although it is presently experiencing transition and change from past configurations. It is not my intention to enter this debate, but only to suggest that if there is a crisis, it is fundamentally a moral one. Our most basic problem is that we are no longer sure what we are doing when we have children or how we should raise them.

It is an irony that there is no better example of this than Kenneth Keniston's *All Our Children*, (Keniston 1977) a book prepared by the Carnegie Council on the Family with the express interest of ensuring the continued strength of the family in our society. Keniston and his colleagues conclude that the family simply cannot be, if it ever was, a self-sufficient unit, and thus argue that all families today need help in raising their children (Keniston 1977, p. 22). The kind of lives parents are leading, and the lives they are preparing their children to live, are so demanding and complex that parents cannot have–and indeed should not have–traditional kinds of direct supervision of their children. This does not mean, according to Keniston, that parents have no role in the raising of their children. Rather, they have a demanding new role: theirs is now the task of choosing, meeting, talking with, and coordinating the experts, the technology, and the institutions which help bring up their children. The specific work involved is familiar to any parent: consultations with teachers, finding good health care, trying to monitor television watching, and so on. "No longer able to do it all themselves, parents today are in some ways like the executives in a large firm–responsible for the smooth coordination of the many people and processes that must work together to produce the final product" (Keniston 1977, p. 17).

I have no interest in trying to deny the descriptive power of Keniston's new understanding of parental responsibility, but at the same time what strikes one is the moral vacuousness of this vision of the family. The idea of the parent as an executive hardly does justice to the kind of commitment we saw exemplified by the parents of retarded children. Indeed, exactly what makes those parents so impressive is their willingness to challenge our society and the "experts" on grounds that they, as parents, know better that their children should not be abandoned by subjecting them to the limits of our technology. Interestingly, Gliedman and Roth's study of discrimination against handicapped children in our society was part of the same Carnegie study as Keniston. It would seem that the underwriting of the rearing of children by professionals recommended by Keniston would be exactly the kind of strategy that Gliedman and Roth find so disastrous for handicapped children. They are clearly aware of this but try to maintain a consistency with Keniston's metaphor of parents as executives by suggesting that parents "must have power–the kind of power that comes with occupying a position of administrative authority in a large organization. Without it, even the best intentioned attempts to reform the way professionals deliver their services risk frustration. For most people–all but the most wealthy, clever, and influential–this power must spring from the same source as that of the administrator–the group. Perhaps more than anything else, it is essential that parents of handicapped children organize themselves into self-help groups" (Gliedman and Roth 1979, pp. 123- 124).

While I am certainly not against "self-help groups," I think that such a suggestion is hardly sufficient to balance what is in effect the moral abdication of parents warranted by Keniston's recommendation. Indeed at a more profound level, I think there is a great difficulty with Gliedman and Roth's attempt to frame the issue of the discrimination against handicapped children as a civil rights issue. For to put the issue that way makes it appear that "handicapped children" are an "oppressed minority" who are independent of their parents. Yet this is exactly what they are not. In fairness to Gliedman and Roth, however, one can easily understand their resort to a civil rights appeal in as much as there appears to be no other moral categories that would suggest why our society should underwrite the attempt of parents to secure adequate care for their retarded children.

But the very moral presuppositions, i.e., assumptions about rights and equality, implied by the language of civil rights fails to give expression to the profound moral commitments involved in parents' struggles to care for their retarded children. For example, we often assume that to be treated equally is to be treated justly, but on reflection we discover that is not the case. For often the language of equality, especially in our society, only works by reducing us to a common denominator, which can be repressive or disrespectful. This can be seen clearly in terms of blacks' struggle for civil rights. This struggle began with a justified call to be treated equally, to have the opportunity to enjoy the same rights of all Americans that blacks were denied on the basis of color. But black Americans soon discovered that it was not enough to be treated equally if that treatment meant they must forget what it means to be black. For who they are as blacks represents a history that should be cherished and enhanced. No one wants to pay the price of being treated equally if that means they must reject who they are-that is, if they must lose their roots in the process of becoming "free" or "equal."

The commitment of parents to their retarded children in this respect involves a more profound and richer sense of community than the language of equality can provide. For the retarded call us toward a community of diversity and difference where that difference is not used as the basis of arbitrary discrimination. (For a fuller account of this point see *Community and Diversity* in this volume.) In this sense, the retarded are a concrete test of the moral implications of a society's willingness to let the differences occasioned by our familial heritages flourish. A society that takes seriously the commitment to the family as the civilizing agency for the rearing of children is one that has learned that equality must not occasion policies that force us to forget or hide our differences–indeed, even the differences that result from being retarded–help each of us to flourish.

But there should be no mistake about it: such a community and society that thrives on differences is a hard enterprise to sustain. We are creatures who fear differences. The fact that the other is not as we are is more often perceived as a threat than as a gift. The only solution is to make others as much like ourselves as possible, or to make them live apart from us, or if necessary, not to live at all. Thus, whites fear blacks, men fear women, and all of us fear the retarded.

Only when we realize this have we reached the point where we can understand the depth of the dilemma raised by our commitment to care for the retarded by and through their parents. Our problem is that we have no philosophy of public morality through which we are able to articulate the kind of commitment we find witnessed in the lives of parents who have learned through their children to be parents. I do not think there is any easy solution to this problem. Rather, I think what we must do is let the witness of such parents guide our way, as they stand as a beacon to remind us what it means to be a parent no matter what our child may he like.

But that they are witnesses only indicates the tenuousness of our situation. How long can we expect to be graced with such presence when we even lack the moral language to express the commitments their lives display? Perhaps, however, in the interim the best thing we can do is to make public these remarkable, but no less ordinary, families.

REFERENCES

Brown, Helene. (1976). *Yesterday's Child.* New York: Signet Books.

Darling, Rosalyn. (1979). *Families Against Society.* Beverly Hills, California: Sage Library of Social Research.

Gliedman, John and Roth, William. (1980). *The Unexpected Minority: Handicapped Children in America.* New York: Harcourt Brace Jovanovich.

Hauerwas, Stanley. (1981). *A Community of Character: Toward a Constructive Christian Social Ethic.* Notre Dame: University of Notre Dame Press.

Keniston, Kenneth. (1977). *All Our Children: The American Family Under Pressure.* New York: Harcourt Brace Jovanovich.

Response to Chapters 9 and 10:
On the Significance of Caring

Linda L. Treloar, PhD, RN, GNP-BC, ANP-C

SUMMARY. The author provides a response to "The Retarded, Society, and the Family: The Dilemma of Care," in which Stanley Hauerwas attempts to establish a moral framework for parenting through observing the actions of parents with children having intellectual disabilities. Treloar's comments on the contemporary situation of caregivers emerge from her perspectives within nursing, disability studies, and perhaps most importantly, experience as the parent of a child (now a young adult) with physical disabilities. *[Article copies available for a fee from The Haworth Document Delivery Service: 1-800-HAWORTH. E-mail address: <docdelivery@haworthpress.com> Website: <http://www.HaworthPress.com> © 2004 by The Haworth Press, Inc. All rights reserved.]*

KEYWORDS. Disability, family, health, caregiving, moral

Dr. Linda L. Treloar, teaches nursing and practices as a geriatric/adult nurse practitioner in Scottsdale, Arizona, USA. She has a PhD in Disability Studies and Health Care Ethics, with research interests in disability, spirituality, and health. Linda is a parent of a young adult daughter with physical disabilities secondary to neuromuscular disease (E-mail: Linda.treloar@sccmail.maricopa.edu).

[Haworth co-indexing entry note]: "Response to Chapters 9 and 10: On the Significance of Caring." Treloar, Linda L. Co-published simultaneously in *Journal of Religion, Disability & Health* (The Haworth Pastoral Press, an imprint of The Haworth Press, Inc.) Vol. 8, No. 3/4, 2004, pp. 181-190; and: *Critical Reflections on Stanley Hauerwas' Theology of Disability: Disabling Society, Enabling Theology* (ed: John Swinton) The Haworth Pastoral Press, an imprint of The Haworth Press, Inc., 2004, pp. 181-190. Single or multiple copies of this article are available for a fee from The Haworth Document Delivery Service [1-800-HAWORTH, 9:00 a.m. - 5:00 p.m. (EST). E-mail address: docdelivery@haworthpress.com].

http://www.haworthpress.com/web/JRDH
© 2004 by The Haworth Press, Inc. All rights reserved.
Digital Object Identifier: 10.1300/J095v8n03_20

Hauerwas attempts to establish a moral framework for parenting through observing the actions of parents with disabled children. His premise is that parents of children with intellectual disabilities, through meeting the needs of their children, are "trained to be parents in a manner that illumines what it means morally to be a parent for anyone." Although the research findings he cites and the language he uses to refer to people with disabilities are dated, the paper remains relevant despite the passage of approximately twenty years. Hauerwas discusses parenting of children with disabilities amid numerous challenges and conflicts posed by helping professionals with non-mutual goals and expectations, a public that fears difference, and a society that lacks a moral consensus that might inform expectations for child care by parents and appropriate governmental assistance to support that care. While Hauerwas' paper focuses on issues surrounding parents and children with intellectual disabilities, his ideas can be applied to families having children with other serious disabilities. My comments emerge from my background within nursing, disability studies, and perhaps most importantly, my experience as the parent of a child (now a young adult) with physical disabilities. Using these three perspectives to reflect on Hauerwas' thinking, I hope to re-contextualise his work and begin to draw out some of its implications for the contemporary situation of carers.

EXPECTATIONS FOR PARENTING

Hauerwas is correct in stating that liberal societies such as the United States, which have a strong foundation for individual human rights, support a person's right to become a parent, irrespective of "the kind of person and thus parent we may be or become." People assume their skills are inherently adequate for parenting. Such thinking of course anticipates the birth of a "normal" child, i.e., one who is not disabled. Having a child with a disability precipitates a redefinition of a parent's image and expectations for the child, and also themselves as individuals, parents, marital partners, and members of a culture and society. This transformational process raises some significant issues which often pass unnoticed. Although many factors influence people's perceptions and behavior toward one another, Hauerwas suggests that others "keep the retarded and their parents at arms length because their presence raises a question most of us prefer remain unasked–namely, what commitments are involved in being a parent that seems to require we care for these children?" In other words: Why do parents choose to care for children with serious intellectual disabilities when this entails great personal expense, and apparent minimal reward?

Perceptions of Disability

Our perceptions surrounding disability are influenced by centuries old beliefs involving stereotype, stigma, and devaluation (Marinelli & Orto, 1999). Too often, we fear and avoid that which we don't understand. Despite current perspectives on disability that view difference as an expected part of the human condition, disability provokes primal conflicts between weakness and strength, dependence and independence, problem and challenge. The occurrence of disability in a family member forces us to examine our implicit and explicit views of the world, stimulating a change in attitudes and behavior, and forcing us to reassess our beliefs about the meaning for disability. As Ted, the father of a child with disabilities put it:

> What has grown for me is an area of compassion . . . being more sensitive to people who are disabled, or not as attractive of mind or body. My sensitivity to their worth and their beauty has increased significantly. When I was in grade school, I was one of those jerks who went out of his way to be mean to kids that couldn't keep up. I've had to do some major rethinking about that. God is a god of concern for everybody; not just people who are 100% physical, 100% mental, 100% anything. (Treloar, 1999b, p. 128)

Disability remains poorly understood by the public. Ridicule and other rejecting behaviors toward people with disabilities exist alongside genuine integration where all persons are seen to have value. Attitudes change through positive encounters between disabled and non-disabled persons, especially when the person we love is disabled. Hauerwas comments: "It is only through intense day-to-day interaction with their children that parents find the means to challenge and change their own stereotypes of what it means to be handicapped as well as find the means to challenge the stereotypes of our society." This is a crucial point. It is this unexplainable ability to see their children as "whole" people that propels parents to advocate for their children, at times appearing to demand care or resources that others see as impractical.

The Family as Caregiver: Conflicts in Caring

Legally and morally, parents are accorded rights to direct their children's care, based on the assumption that they act in the child's best interests. However, as Hauerwas points out, parental obligation to care provides insufficient support for determining the *kind* of care parents should provide. Continuing advances in medical technology and its costs contribute to conflicts over *how much* and *what kind of care is reasonable or appropriate*, and *where care* is given. Hauerwas' thesis is that the family should care for children, both "normal and retarded" in contrast with placing their children who are disabled in institutional settings. Today, deinstitutionalization and the "community imperative" movements insure that children with serious disabilities are no longer preferentially cared for in institutionalized settings. Whenever possible, children remain with their families.

Numerous books, including research-based texts for professionals (e.g., Olkin, 1999; Seligman & Darling, 1997), parent narratives (e.g., Klein & Schive, 2001; Nelson, 1999), and parenting self-help guides (e.g., Fuller & Jones, 1997; Hoekstra & Bradford, 2000; Miller, 1994; Naseef, 1997) herald the benefits and challenges of families who care for children with disabilities. This literature reflects a paradigm shift in how families with disabled children are viewed. Social construction and minority models for disability that view difference as normative, have replaced a historical emphasis on frameworks of mourning, stress, and family dysfunction in families with disabled children (Hanline, 1991). Previous family research anticipated and found pathology, reflecting a medical model for disability that emphasized personal deficits and dysfunction. Contemporary perspectives for disability extend beyond functional impairments, focusing on the environment and its adaptive suitability. Newer family research suggests that the lives of families with disabled children resemble those of other families, exhibiting variability comparable to the general population with respect to important outcomes such as parenting stress, family function, and marital satisfaction (Ferguson, Gartner, & Lipsky, 2000; Krauss, 1993). Parent narratives reveal positive growth, love, and other benefits that support this shift in findings; together with challenges in daily living that are special to, and complicated by disability.

Commonly, at least in the United States, families discover that neither governmental social support nor private health plans offer adequate community-based or in-home assistance for children with high intensity medical needs or disabilities (i.e., autism) that require twenty-four hours a day supervision and care. According to one nurse who works in a state clinic for children with developmental disabilities, doctors who labor diligently to prolong the lives of premature babies in neonatal intensive care units, "don't have a clue" as to the challenges their families face when these children go home. Families may feel inadequately prepared for the immediate and long term effects of caring for a child with disabilities. In my experience, parents who become overwhelmed with caregiving and other family responsibilities find limited options for assistance. Few families can afford to hire health care workers to come into their homes. Non-licensed ancillary staff, such as a nursing assistant may not have the skills to care for the person with a disability. A licensed nurse, if one can be found, doubles or triples the cost. If the family is poor enough to qualify for state assistance, the number of daily hours of non-skilled help is usually extremely limited (5 or 6 hours per day). Although parents may qualify for a limited number of state funded respite (relief) hours each month, an absence overnight or for several days usually requires that their child go to an institutional setting. Most parents that I know choose not to leave, rather than to place their child in an unfamiliar environment.

Parents who have personal limitations in caring for their child, may face other hurdles. The preference for non-institutional care in the United States is so strong that parents who contemplate placing minor children with serious disabilities outside of their home may face significant opposition by others, including funding sources and disability advocates. This is a strange reversal of Hauerwas' 1982 experience! Sadly, although persons with disabilities commonly complain of bias and intolerance toward them by non-disabled persons, I observe some of them displaying similar behaviors toward parents who choose a group or institutional setting for their children with disabilities. One cannot assume that parents who utilize this kind of setting for care of their child are uncaring, self-centered or weak: The decision to allow others to care for their child may signal the culmination of a long struggle involving guilt and sorrow, overwhelming caregiving responsibilities, and concern over the welfare of the child and that of other family members.

Regardless of where their children receive care, Hauerwas states that parents "learn quickly that from the beginning they must fight for their children," establishing and creating resources where inadequate or no resources exist. Parents complain of exhaustion through protracted "battles" with agencies and bureaucratic systems on behalf of their children. Conflicts abound at multiple levels. For example, parents who opt for a classroom geared to children with intellectual disabilities as opposed to an integrated classroom may face significant resistance from professionals and/or disability advocates. Although no one debates the social and personal benefits of integration, parents of children with disabilities may find that in exchange for an inclusive environment, their children do not receive the special kinds of help and services they previously enjoyed. Unfortunately, agency policies may create inflexibility, rather than increased options for an ideal learning environment.

Challenges for Society:
Societal Images for Disability

Although one can argue that Hauerwas' paper is outdated in some aspects, the challenges he describes remain relevant. Social policy initiatives in many westernized countries that promote equal opportunities for people with disabilities (e.g., Americans With Disabilities Act of 1990) exist concurrently with complaints by persons with disabilities that others fail to see them "as persons." While media representations of images and language surrounding disability appear to be improving (Martin & Catlett, 1999), many people associate negative findings, such as tragedy and/or helplessness, with disability. Strategies including the use of "first person language," not in existence when Hauerwas wrote his paper, aim to minimize bias and reinforce healthy representations of disability (see Blaska, 1993). However, other people with disabilities question the benefit of attempts to change attitudes through language, as reported by one woman: "I don't care what you call me. More importantly, address me by my name. I am a person first. Disability is only one spoke on the wheel of my life" (Treloar, personal communication, 1998).

Hauerwas' leading question, "What commitments are involved in being a parent that seems to require we care for these children?" bears no easy answer. How can we explain the actions of parents who devote themselves to caring for children who appear to be able to give little in return? Put more forcefully we might ask: *How can the sacrificial caring out of love for one another be explained?* Readers are encouraged to reflect on how various religious traditions and different cultures address this profoundly spiritual question. In Judeo-Christian culture, all life is worthy of value. Because God loves us, we are to love and care for others. Although some may argue that the United States is not a "Christian culture," these values influenced our founding fathers and continue to influence social policy and law.

Conflicting Goals and Expectations

Helping professionals sometimes complain that parents "do not get it" when they demand health care for their child that appears to be futile. Psychosocial and spiritual issues surrounding disability influence adaptation, topics few helping professionals are comfortable with or prepared to address (Treloar, 1999a). It's easy to assume that parents are denying their child's disability and its accompanying limitations. On the other hand, parents are their child's best advocates, focusing on "what could be," their gaze undimmed by apparent limitations that accompany disability. So, how can professionals and parents work through divergent goals and expectations?

First, one cannot assume that professional perspectives on health and quality of life represent those of people affected by disability. People who effectively adapt to disability may choose to view difficulties associated with disability differently from those who do not share their experience. Disability changes the way in which persons with disabilities accomplish tasks and meet needs. Accommodation to life's challenges may vary from the ideal situation or professionals' recommendations.

Recognition of the knowledge, values, and resources for both the helping professional and the person affected by a disability produces a shift from an authoritarian relationship to a collaborative and supportive relationship (see The Intersystem Model in Artinian & Conger, 1997). In the beginning, parents benefit from information that explains their child's condition, provides help and support that assists them to accept themselves and their child and provide care for the child, along with guidance and hope for the future. As parents gain skill and confidence in caring for their children, they become the "expert" in the care of their child. Their knowledge rivals that of the professional; they become the "knowledgeable patient/family member" (Treloar & Artinian, 2001). The professional must ask the parent what works best for him or her and what goals are being pursued, assuming a collaborative partnership in the care of the child. Goals and interventions should address disabling environmental and social barriers. Similarly, the knowledgeable adult with a disability will work more effectively with helping professionals who respect him or her and incorporate similar treatment principles.

An interdisciplinary team perspective that places the person/family at its head, and that extends into the community is needed. Professionals should promote self-care and participation in personal health care: We must plan *with*, rather than *for* the person/family. This requires open communication, unrestrained by power and position differences. Consistent with the social model for disability, helping professionals must attempt to alleviate environmental limitations that impair a disabled person's ability to live his/her life to the same extent as a non-disabled person.

Social and Bioethical Challenges

Countries with fewer resources offer limited life-saving and rehabilitative options to parents of children with disabilities. In the United States, medical technology extends the lives of premature babies and disabled persons, both young and old that would not survive in poorer countries. Escalating costs of health care and increasing people in need create competition for finite resources. Countries with life-saving medical technology grapple with questions involving futility: Is all care beneficial? Does the ability to care necessitate its use? How will we determine who receives what resources? For example, in the United States neonatal intensive care units find very low birth weight infants tethered to machines and other life-saving treatments. Although the majority of survivors escape serious disabilities, the cohort of children in one recent study (Hack et al., 2002) experienced higher rates of developmental disabilities and neurological problems that persist into adulthood. In a second example, public school districts in affluent and poor areas alike report budgetary limitations that affect the quality of education (e.g., see Jaquiss, 2002). Although schools receive state funding at a higher level for students with disabilities, seldom are budgets adequate to cover children whose accompanying medical needs (e.g., a child on a ventilator) necessitate the full-time skills of a licensed nurse, for example. How will administrators decide whether the needs of one child, or those of many children take priority? Options for resolving conflicts between parents, professionals, or payor sources include negotiation, legislation, or judicial decisions. Further, the need for hard decisions involving resource allocation will increase as western-ized nations worldwide continue to age.

Final Thoughts

Today, families with disabled children benefit from social policy initiatives and legislation that promote equal opportunities. Large institutions that for-merly housed vast numbers of people with severe intellectual disabilities have been replaced by community-based alternatives. Negative public attitudes to-ward people with disabilities are improving; bias and discrimination may be cloaked, rather than overt. At the same time, conflicts abound at multiple lev-els; often producing a quagmire for people whose lives are affected by disabil-ity.

Parents remain their disabled child's best advocate. Caregivers and persons with disabilities who live "normal" lives continue to be perceived as "heroic." In my experience, most do not see themselves in this way; they are simply do-ing what is needed to live their lives. Perceptual difficulties abound, affecting both people who are touched or untouched by disability. For example, parents and maturing children may experience conflicts associated with individuation and leaving home. Disability complicates the young adult's task of leaving and separation. Based on personal experience and the stories of other families, I doubt that parents and their adult children with disabilities can readily under-stand the perspectives of the other as this relates to parenting decisions.

Can the actions of parents who care for children with serious disabilities provide a moral example for others? One mother's words (Dwight, 2001) il-lustrate Hauerwas' point that children with serious disabilities teach their par-ents how to care for them:

> My first son, Timmy, a strong-willed, inquisitive boy, had taught my husband, Phil, and me many things. . . . But I don't think I came face to face with the true meaning of motherhood until Aidan entered our lives eighteen months ago. (p. 18)

As I poured over the books and talked with these other parents, I found the factual side of Down syndrome fairly easy to piece together. . . . Of course, there was nothing in those reference books that could fully explain the other side of the story–the ups and downs of raising a child with Down syndrome in our society. That's what we've been learning from Aidan himself, and it's been a lesson filled with wonder. . . . We're learning, as all parents discover with the birth of their second child, that each child is different. (pp. 34-35)

In many ways, our lives have been transformed. We have found loving support from people who used to be strangers. We look at the world differently. . . . We have an appreciation for a slower pace. . . . And we have a newfound understanding of the preciousness of all people. (p. 37)

Parenting Aidan, a child with a disability, allowed his mother to experience the "true meaning of motherhood." I agree with Hauerwas (1982) that other parents can learn from the moral example of parental caring she demonstrates. And similar to this mother, I can testify that: Disability changes our world; we will never be the same. Thanks to our children with disabilities for that gift!

REFERENCES

Artinian, B. M., & Conger, M. M. (Eds.) (1997). *The Intersystem Model: Integrating Theory and Practice*. Thousand Oaks, CA: Sage.

Blaska, J. (1993). 'The power of language: Speak and write using "person first."' In M. Nagler (Ed.), *Perspectives on Disability: Text and Readings on Disability* (pp. 25-32). Palo Alto, CA: Health Markets Research.

Dwight, V. (2001). 'Adian's gift.' In S. D. Klein and K. Schive (Eds.), *You Will Dream New Dreams: Inspiring Personal Stories by Parents of Children with Disabilities* (pp. 31-37). New York, NY: Kensington Publishing Corp.

Ferguson, P. M., Gartner, A., & Lipsky, D. K. (2000). 'The experience of disability in families: A synthesis of research and parent narratives.' In E. Parens and A. Asch (Eds.), *Prenatal Testing and Disability Rights* (pp. 72-94). Washington, D.C.: Georgetown University Press.

Fuller, C., & Jones, L. T. (1997). *Extraordinary Kids: Nurturing and Championing Your Child with Special Needs*. Colorado Springs, CO: Focus on the Family Publishing.

Hack, M., Flannery, D. J., Schluchter, M., Cartar, L., Borawski, E., & Klein, N. (2002). 'Outcomes in young adulthood for very-low-birth-weight infants.' *The New England Journal of Medicine, 346*(3), 149-157.

Hanline, M. F. (1991). 'Transitions and critical events in the family life cycle: Implications for providing support to families of children with disabilities.' *Psychology in the Schools, 28*(1), 53-59.

Hauerwas, S. (Ed.) (1982). *Responsibility for Devalued Persons*. Springfield, IL: Charles C. Thomas.

Hoekstra, E., & Bradford, M. (2000). *Chronic Kids: Constant Hope*. Wheaton, IL: Crossway Books.

Jaquiss, N. (2002). *The Crushing Cost of Special Education* (Willamette Week Online), [Electronic version]. Willamette Week Newspaper. Available: http://www.wweek. com/ flatfiles/allstories.lasso?reckie=12603522 [2002, March 13].

Klein, S. D., & Schive, K. (Eds.). (2001). *You Will Dream New Dreams: Inspiring Personal Stories by Parents of Children with Disabilities*. New York: Kensington Publishing Corp.

Krauss, M. W. (1993). 'Child-related and parenting stress: Similarities and differences between mothers and fathers of children with disabilities.' *American Journal on Mental Retardation, 97*(4), 393-404.

Marinelli, R. P., & Orto, A. E. D. (Eds.) (1999). *The Psychological and Social Impact of Disability* (4th ed.). New York: Springer.

Martin, S. S., & Catlett, S. M. (1999). 'Same window, new view: Print media and persons with disabilities.' Unpublished paper presented at 1999 TASH Conference, Chicago, IL.

Miller, N. B. (1994). *Nobody's Perfect: Living and Growing with Children Who Have Special Needs*. Baltimore, MD: Paul H. Brookes Publishing.

Naseef, R. A. (1997). *Special Children, Challenged Parents: The Struggles and Rewards of Raising a Child with a Disability*. Secaucus, NJ: A Birch Lane Press Book, Carol Publishing Group.

Nelson, C. L. (1999). *Eagle Doctor: Stories of Stephen, My Child with Special Needs*. St. Paul, MN: Pangaea.

Olkin, R. (1999). *What Psychotherapists Should Know about Disability*. New York: The Guilford Press.

Seligman, M., & Darling, R. B. (1997). *Ordinary Families, Special Children: A Systems Approach to Childhood Disability* (2nd ed.). New York: Guilford Press.

Treloar, L. L. (1999a). 'People with disabilities–The same, but different: Implications for health care practice.' *Journal of Transcultural Nursing, 10*(4), 358-364.

Treloar, L. L. (1999b). *Perceptions of Spiritual Beliefs, Response to Disability, and the Church*. Unpublished Doctoral dissertation [listed in Dissertation Abstracts International, Vol/Issue 60-02A, University Microfilms International No. AAI9919753, p. 562], The Union Institute and University, Cincinnati, OH.

Treloar, L. L., & Artinian, B. (2001). Chapter 19: Populations Affected by Disabilities. In M. A. Nies & M. McEwen (Eds.), *Community Health Nursing: Promoting the Health of Aggregates* (3rd ed., pp. 496-525). Philadelphia: W.B. Saunders.

Chapter 11

Reflection on Dependency:
A Response to Responses
to My Essays on Disability

Stanley Hauerwas, PhD

SUMMARY. In this final chapter Hauerwas responds to the papers that have been presented within this volume. *[Article copies available for a fee from The Haworth Document Delivery Service: 1-800-HAWORTH. E-mail address: <docdelivery@haworthpress.com> Website: <http://www.HaworthPress.com> © 2004 by The Haworth Press, Inc. All rights reserved.]*

KEYWORDS. Disability, theology, community, liberal society

DISABILITY THEOLOGICALLY CONSIDERED

I am extremely grateful to John Swinton for conceiving this book and to those who have responded to the individual essays. It never occurred to me that the essays I have written over the years about disability, and in particular that kind of disability labeled "mental," might be fruitfully brought together. The responses to the various essays, at least for me, are what justifies this col-

---

[Haworth co-indexing entry note]: "Reflection on Dependency: A Response to Responses to My Essays on Disability." Hauerwas, Stanley. Co-published simultaneously in *Journal of Religion, Disability & Health* (The Haworth Pastoral Press, an imprint of The Haworth Press, Inc.) Vol. 8, No. 3/4, 2004, pp. 191-197; and: *Critical Reflections on Stanley Hauerwas' Theology of Disability: Disabling Society, Enabling Theology* (ed: John Swinton) The Haworth Pastoral Press, an imprint of The Haworth Press, Inc., 2004, pp. 191-197. Single or multiple copies of this article are available for a fee from The Haworth Document Delivery Service [1-800-HAWORTH, 9:00 a.m. - 5:00 p.m. (EST). E-mail address: docdelivery@haworthpress.com].

http://www.haworthpress.com/web/JRDH
Digital Object Identifier: 10.1300/J095v8n03_21

lection of my essays. I am, therefore, in debt to those who have given me the gift of criticism of the essays I have written on disability.

However that those that responded wrote on a specific essay or a selection of essays creates a difficulty if I try to respond to each of the reactions to my various essays. I hope, for example, it will be obvious that some of the criticism directed at particular essays is at least anticipated and responded to in other essays in the book. For example I have been and continue to be acutely aware of the problem of "labeling" the mentally handicapped, but I do not discuss that problem in every essay in this book. I will return to the problem of descriptions we use to characterize what is taken to be "the problem" of the mentally handicapped, but I hope readers of this book will notice that I begin to respond to some of the criticism of a particular essay in other essays collected in this book.

Accordingly, I will not try to respond to every point made by those who have written essays in this book. Assuming a defensive posture strikes me as self-defeating for what I and my responders care about. This is no place to score intellectual points. The topic we are considering is far too important for academic game play. What we care about is helping ourselves and others think through what it means to learn to be with the mentally handicapped. What is at stake in this discussion is not this or that theoretical position, but rather how to protect those we have come to love from threats to their very existence ironically justified by appeals to the highest "ideals" of our culture. If this book does not in some way help us better be loved by and to love those labeled "mentally handicapped," I will be (as I am sure those who responded to these essays will be) severely disappointed.

This brings me to the question I raise in the essay, "Timeful Friends: Living with the Handicapped," namely: Have I "used" the mentally handicapped in support of theological and ethical arguments in a manner that is unjustified? I have certainly "used" the "mentally handicapped" to explore theological questions that may not be first and foremost "about" the "handicapped." I have "used" the challenge presented by the mentally handicapped in an effort to show that theological questions are never "just theoretical" but have implications for how we understand our lives as Christians. In doing so I hope what I have done is not a misuse of the handicapped, but rather is a way to draw attention to their significance for any faithful understanding of the church.

One of the frustrating aspects of my work, for friend and foe alike, is I have always tried to do theology by indirection. By indirection I mean I have tried to resist the temptation to make theology another set of ideas that can be considered in and of themselves. For example, anyone concerned to discover what "my" doctrine of God might be or what my "theological anthropology" entails will look in vain for any essay or book on those theological topics. But that does not mean I do not think about questions classically associated with the doctrine of God or theological anthropology; I try to write about such issues in relation to material practices that exemplify what is at stake.

My reflections on the challenge the mentally handicapped present to some of our most cherished conceits about ourselves is best understood as my attempt to develop a theological anthropology. In brief, I "use" the mentally handicapped to try to help us understand what it means for us to be creatures of a gracious God. For I think it a profound mistake to assume that a strong distinction can be drawn between those who are mentally handicapped and those who are not mentally handicapped once it is acknowledged that we are equally creatures of a God, who as Augustine observed, created us without us, but who refuses to save us without us. The mentally handicapped remind us that the "us" that is saved is the body constituted through Christian baptism that is anything but an individual. If we take seriously practices of the church such as baptism, we are all, mentally handicapped and the non-mentally handicapped, creatures drawn into a kingdom of patience making possible our friendship with God and one another.

I do not assume that such a view is peculiar only to Christians. Indeed I think Alasdair MacIntyre in his book, *Dependent Rational Animals: Why Human Beings Need the Virtues* (Chicago: Open Court, 1999) has wonderfully argued that the often drawn strong distinction between humans and animals cannot be justified on philosophical grounds. So I am not surprised, indeed I am delighted, that Michael Bérubé–who does not share my theological convictions–discovers the gift that is his son. Accordingly we are gifted by Michael Bérubé's account of his son, Jamie, as well as by Bérubé's confession that neither he nor his wife could sustain his son's life by themselves. They need help, which is but a reminder that that is who we are–creatures who need help. We desperately need one another, but if we forget or deny such need, we cannot help but become less than we were meant to be.

I need to be very clear when I am making these kinds of observations that I am not suggesting that the existence of the mentally handicapped is justified because they make us better people by demanding our care of them. Though it is certainly the case that some of us are made better because of the call of those identified as mentally handicapped, that is not a reason to justify their existence. Their existence does not need to be justified–which is but a reminder that no one's existence needs to be justified. I exist, you exist, Jamie exists, turtles exist, the earth exists by the grace of God. The task is to learn to rejoice in our existence without resentment.

I have engaged in a polemic with the ideologies and practices of modernity that tempt us to forget the "giftedness" of our existence. Christopher Newell's observation that he has never met a utilitarian with a disability is a pungent comment that reveals the inhumanity that is often hidden in humanistic presumptions. Of course, it is not just the philosophical positions so prominent in our time that threaten the mentally handicapped, but the political and economic arrangements that to a greater or lesser extent institutionalize those philosophical presumptions. Whether we like it or not–and I confess I wish it were not so–the mentally handicapped, like the canary used by miners in a mine, help us spot the "gas" in our lives that threatens our humanity.

So I cannot deny that I have "used" the mentally handicapped to develop my contention that if we are to make sense of their existence and our existence with them, it surely makes equal sense that the God Christians worship is in fact the God who moves the sun and the stars and our hearts. My project has always been to help Christians ask what kind of people we need to be, what kind of practices should constitute our lives, to be able to welcome children into our lives some of whom may be born "different." I am appreciative that several who responded to my essays thought I did not manipulate the disabled for my personal ends, but they could have well accused me of using the disabled for theological ends. I surely must plead guilty that I have "used" the mentally handicapped to help us see why, if the mentally handicapped matter, then what Christians believe about the way things are matters. I hope, however, I have tried to do no more than to witness to the witness that Jean Vanier is.

I admire Michael Bérubé's attempt to sustain a modest humanism. I have every reason to join him in the effort to maintain such a humanism. So I welcome Bérubé's desire to be a presence for Christians as we are hopefully a presence for him. For he knows far too well that in our time it has proven to be very difficult to maintain such a modest humanism. In the name of the good of "mankind" intolerable evils are perpetrated. Jamie rightly asks his father to "always be my friend," and may that friendship make possible friendships that can serve to stand against those who would rather the Jamies not exist. Which is but my way of saying to Berube how deeply I was moved by his response to my article.

I find it difficult, however, to engage polemically Aileen Barclay's response to my essay "The Gesture of a Truthful Story." She is quite right that her response does reveal her "liberal roots," but she is quite wrong to identify me as a "traditional evangelical." If I am anything I am a "traditional Catholic" which means I seldom talk about "lived experience." (It is an interesting question to ask what would count as an "unlived experience.") However, I owe her some clarifications that I hope will help her and others who may share her commitments to understand the differences between us.

I would never make a generalization about the "world religions" because I think the very notion of religion is problematic. That does not mean I think Christianity is superior to other ways of life, because such a judgment presumes epistemological presumptions I think are deeply problematic. The distinction between church and world is not an epistemological distinction, but reflects the eschatological commitments that are at the heart of the Gospel. If Barclay has a problem with a dichotomous division between church and world, I simply have to suggest it is not me with whom she is in disagreement but the New Testament and, in particular, the Gospel of John. The focus on the mentally handicapped is but a way to help us make the distinction between church and world concrete. The world names all those who are aware of a world of agony and cannot take the time, the patience, to care for those who will not get "better." Of course it is the same world that may well produce people like the Bérubés, who remind Christians of our profoundest convictions.

I have no reason to deny that the distinction between church and world is open to abuse, but what is not open to abuse? Yet there is nothing about that distinction that would legitimate the withdrawal of the church from the world, but rather the distinction helps name the way the church must be in the world. For example, we live in a world of impatience, a world that thrives on speed, a world that values efficiency above all things. If the church is to be a community that is constituted by sharing our lives with the mentally handicapped, then the church's patience cannot help but be a contrast to the hurry that is the world. I cannot imagine a more important witness the church has for such a hurried world.

So I am sympathetic to Ray Anderson's worry about my suggestion that we should be willing to have our medical practice as fragmented as our lives, but I was not making a recommendation. Rather I was simply trying to help us see that that already is the way things are; but we have trouble seeing that is the way things are if there does not exist an alternative community with alternative practices. Again the church does not wish the world to be worse than it may be in order for the church to "look good." But rather if the church is not faithful, if the church lacks the patience to care for the disabled, then we will lack the resources to describe truthfully the world in which we find ourselves. I am brought back to the issue of labeling.

The Language of Disability, or Why No Description Is Satisfactory

I wish I had, but I do not have, any satisfactory suggestion to make about the problem of labeling the mentally handicapped. Labels not only are derogatory, they also invite self-fulfilling prophecies. Yet it seems some label is needed in order to suggest the interventions that may be helpful. Downs Syndrome will not tell us a great deal about Mary or Billy, but that label can be a helpful shorthand for those who want to help Mary or Billy to flourish. Of course, what the description, Downs Syndrome, suggests will need to be constantly tested through the ongoing work with people so described.

I am very sympathetic with those that would like to leave all such descriptions behind. But in the attempt to recommend they be left behind, we too often use the very description we are trying to leave behind–e.g., we should no longer use a phrase like mentally handicapped to describe the mentally handicapped. I remember well the time I was challenged at a conference by a wonderful lady who had cerebral palsy that I should not use the description "retarded." She spoke in solidarity with the mentally handicapped, but she was able to do so because her disability did not disable her speech. I provide this example only because I know of no way to avoid descriptions that may distort the life of some.

The issue, of course, is not just the label, but who gets to use the label. Unfortunately the label is too often used by some to secure power over others in the name of being "helpful." That is why it is so important that forms of "care" be given in communities in which the care giver understands that the one being cared for is giving a gift of vulnerability. This is not only true of relations between the disabled and those that care for the disabled, but occurs every time a patient presents their body to a physician. "Assistants" in L'Arche houses have the advantage that the liturgy reminds them on a daily basis that those they assist are giving them a gift. When the liturgy is not at the heart of such giving and receiving labels, will always be as dangerous as they are helpful.

Only names can defeat labels. If Boyce is first and foremost Boyce, then he can never be just another "Downs." So I worry a bit about Jean Vanier's suggestion that a distinction can be drawn between basic needs and those needs which allow a person to flourish. The needs identified with flourishing, e.g., love, respect, dignity, and friendship, I suspect are often embodied in food, lodging, education, and medical help. That is to say, if we rightly call Boyce by his name, we should be very careful not to separate his basic needs from his call of love to us. I agree entirely with Christopher Newell's suggestion that we need to learn to talk with the disabled rather than to talk at them. But such an accomplishment surely depends on our knowing that their name tells us more about them than any disability they may suffer.

This is the main reason I find it hard to write any longer about the mentally handicapped. I no longer know sufficiently the names of people who are handicapped. I do not trust myself to write truthfully about those I do not know. In such a circumstance I fear I really will be using those whose names I do not know for purposes they cannot own. I do, however, find it encouraging that in some of the responses, those who work with the disabled find at least some of what I have done helpful for them to voice their understanding of what they do.

I am but reminding us that more important than my theological reflections on the handicapped are the stories written by parents and friends of the handicapped. Those stories are necessary to break the silence that too often isolates us from one another, making friendship impossible. Without such narratives, suffering can too quickly become an invitation to narcissism. Without shared narratives, we can lose the joy that comes from the simple tasks that make life between ourselves and the disabled possible.

Speech is crucial for our relationship to one another; but speech can become just noise that drowns out appropriate silence. The language of gesture is my attempt to remind us of the significance of the body whose silence often tells us what we most need to know to be with one another. Professor Swinton suggests that the focus on gestures as well as the emphasis on the contextual character of truth seem to imply that I assume gestures are non-cognitive. I can understand why the language of gesture may be so interpreted, but for me gestures entail the most determinative cognitive claims we can make. They do so because the claims so made cannot be abstracted from the ones making the claim. The disabled are but reminders that before God none of us are whole; but God makes possible the joining of our bodies through which we become whole.

Who I Hope Will Read This Book

I love John O'Brien's suggestion that in the article, "Community and Diversity: Living With the Handicapped" my pronouns keep "sliding around." O'Brien notes that this makes it hard to know for whom I am writing. The answer is I am writing for those that do not yet exist. Of course, many parents and care givers read my essays as initiated "insiders." I hope to be taught by them in what ways I am getting these matters right or wrong. But the "you" that is the primary focus of these essays is you I hope discover that they are part of a community they had not noticed. Once discovering they are so situated, I hope that their Christian practices and convictions begin to feel strange and yet more real.

So I hope this book may attract readers who have never had to think about or deal with the disabled. For this is not a book to be read only by those who have already been drawn into the world of disability. It is a book for Christians, but I hope non-Christians may find in these pages a discussion that suggests a different kind of Christianity than they normally encounter. For here we see a people who believe there is nothing more significant to be done in a world of such deep injustice than to take the time to be friends with the handicapped. I know of no better vision of peace.

Index